Evolving Role of PET in Assessing the Efficacy of Immunotherapy and Radiation Therapy in Malignant Disorders

Editors

CHARLES B. SIMONE II
NICOLAS AIDE
ABASS ALAVI

PET CLINICS

www.pet.theclinics.com

Consulting Editor
ABASS ALAVI

January 2020 • Volume 15 • Number 1

ELSEVIER

1600 John F. Kennedy Boulevard • Suite 1800 • Philadelphia, Pennsylvania, 19103-2899

http://www.pet.theclinics.com

PET CLINICS Volume 15, Number 1
January 2020 ISSN 1556-8598, ISBN-13: 978-0-323-71072-5

Editor: John Vassallo (j.vassallo@elsevier.com)
Developmental Editor: Casey Potter

PET Clinics (ISSN 1556-8598) is published quarterly by Elsevier Inc., 360 Park Avenue South, New York, NY 10010-1710. Months of issue are January, April, July, and October. Periodicals postage paid at New York, NY, and additional mailing offices. Subscription prices per year are $247.00 (US individuals), $422.00 (US institutions), $100.00 (US students), $279.00 (Canadian individuals), $475.00 (Canadian institutions), $100.00 (Canadian students), $275.00 (foreign individuals), $475.00 (foreign institutions), and $140.00 (foreign students). To receive student and resident rate, orders must be accompanied by name of affiliated institution, date of term, and the signature of program/residency coordinator on institution letterhead. Orders will be billed at individual rate until proof of status is received. Foreign air speed delivery is included in all Clinics subscription prices. All prices are subject to change without notice. POSTMASTER: Send address changes to PET Clinics, Elsevier Health Sciences Division, Subscription Customer Service, 3251 Riverport Lane, Maryland Heights, MO 63043. **Customer Service: 1-800-654-2452 (U.S. and Canada); 314-447-8871 (outside U.S. and Canada). Fax: 314-447-8029. E-mail: journalscustomerservice-usa@elsevier.com (for print support); journalsonlinesupport-usa@elsevier.com (for online support).**

Reprints. For copies of 100 or more of articles in this publication, please contact the Commercial Reprints Department, Elsevier Inc., 360 Park Avenue South, New York, NY 10010-1710. Tel.: 212-633-3874; Fax: 212-633-3820; E-mail: reprints@elsevier.com.

Printed in the United States of America.

PET Clinics is covered in MEDLINE/PubMed (Index Medicus).

Contributors

CONSULTING EDITOR

ABASS ALAVI, MD, MD (Hon), PhD (Hon), DSc (Hon)
Professor of Radiology, Division of Nuclear Medicine, Department of Radiology, Hospital of the University of Pennsylvania, University of Pennsylvania Perelman School of Medicine, Philadelphia, Pennsylvania, USA

EDITORS

CHARLES B. SIMONE II, MD
Department of Radiation Oncology, New York Proton Center, New York, New York, USA

NICOLAS AIDE, MD, PhD
Professor, Service de Médecine Nucléaire, CHU de CAEN, Avenue Côte de Nacre, Caen, France; Full Professor of Nuclear Medicine of the Caen University Hospital, University of Normandy, France

ABASS ALAVI, MD, MD (Hon), PhD (Hon), DSc (Hon)
Professor of Radiology, Division of Nuclear Medicine, Department of Radiology, Hospital of the University of Pennsylvania, University of Pennsylvania Perelman School of Medicine, Philadelphia, Pennsylvania, USA

AUTHORS

ERIK H.J.G. AARNTZEN, MD, PhD
Department of Radiology and Nuclear Medicine, Radboud University Medical Center, Nijmegen, The Netherlands

TONY ABRAHAM, DO, MPA
Department of Radiology (Nuclear Medicine), Albert Einstein College of Medicine, Bronx, New York, USA

NICOLAS AIDE, MD, PhD
Professor, Service de Médecine Nucléaire, CHU de CAEN, Avenue Côte de Nacre, Caen, France; Full Professor of Nuclear Medicine of the Caen University Hospital, University of Normandy, France

ABASS ALAVI, MD, MD (Hon), PhD (Hon), DSc (Hon)
Professor of Radiology, Division of Nuclear Medicine, Department of Radiology, Hospital of the University of Pennsylvania, University of Pennsylvania Perelman School of Medicine, Philadelphia, Pennsylvania, USA

SANDIP BASU, MBBS (Hons), DRM, Diplomate N.B., MNAMS
Radiation Medicine Centre (BARC), Tata Memorial Hospital Annexe, Homi Bhabha National Institute, Mumbai, India

N. PATRIK BRODIN, PhD
Institute for Onco-Physics, Albert Einstein College of Medicine, Department of Radiation Oncology, Montefiore Medical Center, Bronx, New York, USA

JASON W. CHAN, MD
Department of Radiation Oncology, Helen Diller Family Comprehensive Cancer Center, University of California, San Francisco, San Francisco, California, USA

MICHAEL CHUONG, MD
Department of Radiation Oncology, Miami
Cancer Institute, Miami, Florida, USA

ALEXANDRA D. DREYFUSS, BS
Department of Radiology, Hospital of the
University of Pennsylvania, University of
Pennsylvania, Philadelphia, Pennsylvania, USA

CHUNXIAO GUO, MD
Department of Interventional Radiology, The
University of Texas MD Anderson Cancer
Center, Houston, Texas, USA

SANDRA HESKAMP, MD, PhD
Department of Radiology and Nuclear
Medicine, Radboud University Medical Center,
Nijmegen, The Netherlands

RODNEY J. HICKS, MD, FRACP
Director of Molecular Imaging and Therapeutic
Nuclear Medicine, Cancer Imaging, The Peter
MacCallum Cancer Centre, Melbourne,
Victoria, Australia

NICOLE A. HOHENSTEIN, BA
Department of Radiation Oncology, Helen
Diller Family Comprehensive Cancer Center,
University of California, San Francisco, San
Francisco, California, USA

AMIR IRAVANI, MD, FRACP
Nuclear Medicine Physician, Cancer Imaging,
The Peter MacCallum Cancer Centre,
Melbourne, Victoria, Australia

PEGAH JAHANGIRI, MD
Department of Radiology, Hospital of the
University of Pennsylvania, University of
Pennsylvania, Philadelphia, Pennsylvania, USA

ADEEL KAISER, MD
Department of Radiation Oncology, University
of Maryland School of Medicine, Baltimore,
Maryland, USA

ANTONY KOROULAKIS, MD
Department of Radiation Oncology, University
of Maryland Medical Center, Baltimore,
Maryland, USA

EGESTA LOPCI, MD, PhD
Nuclear Medicine, Humanitas Clinical and
Research Hospital–IRCCS, Milan, Italy

MICHEL MEIGNAN, MD, PhD
Radiology, Lysa Imaging and Haematology,
Hôpitaux Universitaires Henri Mondor,
Henri Mondor University Hospitals,
Créteil, France

HARI MENON, BS
University of Arizona College of Medicine,
Phoenix, Arizona, USA

JASON K. MOLITORIS, MD, PhD
Department of Radiation Oncology, University
of Maryland School of Medicine, Baltimore,
Maryland, USA

NITIN OHRI, MD
Institute for Onco-Physics, Albert Einstein
College of Medicine, Department of Radiation
Oncology, Montefiore Medical Center, Bronx,
New York, USA

RAHUL V. PARGHANE, MBBS, MD
Radiation Medicine Centre (BARC), Tata
Memorial Hospital Annexe, Homi Bhabha
National Institute, Mumbai, India

BERBER PIET, MD
Department of Pulmonary Diseases, Radboud
University Medical Center, Nijmegen, The
Netherlands

KEVIN PRIGENT, MD, MS
Resident, Nuclear Medicine Department,
University Hospital, Service de Médecine
Nucléaire, CHU de CAEN, Caen,
France

STEPHANIE R. RICE, MD
Department of Radiation Oncology, University
of Maryland Medical Center, Baltimore,
Maryland, USA

SHAHNEEN SANDHU, MBBS, FRACP
Medical Oncologist, Department of Oncology,
The Peter MacCallum Cancer Centre,
Melbourne, Victoria, Australia

ANKUR M. SHARMA, MD
Department of Radiation Oncology, Maryland
Proton Treatment Center, University of
Maryland School of Medicine, Baltimore,
Maryland, USA; Harvard T.H. Chan School of
Public Health, Harvard University, Boston,
Massachusetts, USA

OSMAN M. SIDDIQUI, MD
Department of Radiation Oncology, University of Maryland Medical Center, Baltimore, Maryland, USA

CHARLES B. SIMONE II, MD
Department of Radiation Oncology, New York Proton Center, New York, New York, USA

PEGGY TAHIR, MA, MLIS
UCSF Library, University of California, San Francisco, San Francisco, California, USA

WOLFGANG A. TOMÉ, PhD
Institute for Onco-Physics, Albert Einstein College of Medicine, Department of Radiation Oncology, Montefiore Medical Center, Department of Neurology, Albert Einstein College of Medicine, Bronx, New York, USA

MICHEL M. VAN DEN HEUVEL, MD, PhD
Department of Pulmonary Diseases, Radboud University Medical Center, Nijmegen, The Netherlands

CARLA M.L. VAN HERPEN, MD, PhD
Department of Medical Oncology, Radboud University Medical Center, Nijmegen, The Netherlands

SARAH R. VERHOEFF, MD
Department of Medical Oncology, Radboud University Medical Center, Nijmegen, The Netherlands

VIVEK VERMA, MD
Department of Radiation Oncology, Allegheny General Hospital, Pittsburgh, Pennsylvania, USA

SUSAN Y. WU, MD
Department of Radiation Oncology, Helen Diller Family Comprehensive Cancer Center, University of California, San Francisco, San Francisco, California, USA

SUE S. YOM, MD, PhD, MAS
Department of Radiation Oncology, Helen Diller Family Comprehensive Cancer Center, University of California, San Francisco, San Francisco, California, USA

Contents

After a short summary of the biological basis of the immune checkpoint inhibitors used for the treatment of nonhematologic solid tumors, the issues of pseudoprogression, hyperprogression, and immune-related side effects are discussed as well as their implications for patient management. Recommendations are provided for performing ^{18}F-Fludeoxyglucose PET scanning, assessing tumor response, and reporting immune-related side effects, with representative clinical cases.

The complexity of the immune response and diversity of targets challenges conventional conceptual frameworks used in selecting and monitoring treatment with immune check-point inhibitors. The limitations of anatomic imaging in assessing response have been recognized. Varying patterns of response have been recognized. These patterns have different implications for the continuation and duration of therapy. Evidence supporting the role of ^{18}F-fluorodeoxyglucose Positron Emission Tomography/Computed Tomography as a prognostic biomarker and in characterizing response is presented. An added benefit of this approach is the ability to detect immune-related inflammatory reactions, often in advance of severe or life-threatening clinical manifestations.

Response assessment in malignant lymphoma has progressively evolved in the last 20 years, leading to continuous adaptations to clinical requirements and technology improvements. The latest challenge in treatment evaluation is represented by immunomodulatory drugs, capable of stimulating response to cancer by unleashing the immune system of the host. Despite the consolidated consensus on the use of Deauville score and Lugano criteria for the assessment of first-line therapeutic regimens, during other lines of treatment and, particularly, during the course of immunotherapy, response parameters and clinical evidence appear less clear.

Clinical indications for immune checkpoint inhibitor (ICI) therapy are rapidly expanding for various stages of several solid tumors. The success of ICIs results from a complex interplay between cancer cells and their immune microenvironment. PD-1/PD-L1 PET imaging enables to study of these interactions in the tumor microenvironment in a clinical setting. These noninvasive, sensitive and quantitative tools may play an important role in optimizing ICI efficacy.

monitoring in colorectal and anal malignancies. Use of PET/CT for GI malignancies continues to evolve over time, with new studies evaluating prognostic abilities of PET/CT and with increasing sensitivity and spatial resolution of more modern PET/CT scanners. The authors encourage future applications and prospective evaluation of the use of PET/CT in the staging, prognostication, and recurrence prediction for GI malignancies.

Evolving Role of Novel Quantitative PET Techniques to Detect Radiation-Induced Complications

Alexandra D. Dreyfuss, Pegah Jahangiri, Charles B. Simone II, and Abass Alavi

Radiation-induced normal tissue toxicities vary in terms of pathophysiologic determinants and timing of disease development, and they are influenced by the dose and radiation volume the critical organs receive, and the radiosensitivity of normal tissues and their baseline rate of cell turnover. Radiation-induced lung injury is dose limiting for the treatment of lung and thoracic cancers and can lead to fibrosis and potentially fatal pneumonitis. This article focuses on pulmonary and cardiovascular complications of radiation therapy and discusses how PET-based novel quantitative techniques can be used to detect these events earlier than current imaging modalities or clinical presentation allow.

PET/Computed Tomography in Treatment Response Assessment in Cancer: An Overview with Emphasis on the Evolving Role in Response Evaluation to Immunotherapy and Radiation Therapy

Rahul V. Parghane and Sandip Basu

The effectiveness of cancer treatment must be assessed early in the course of the therapy so that regimens can be tailored in an individualized manner. Whole-body metabolic burden, metabolic tumor volume and total lesion glycolysis are the newer quantitative PET metrics that reflect the overall disease burden and take into account the stage of the disease, the heterogeneous intra-tumoral metabolism and uptake of PET tracer. Immunotherapy response evaluation in solid tumors is challenging, and combined use of anatomical and molecular imaging could evolve as the optimal way for assessing treatment response to immunotherapy. PET based parameters may be better predictors of response, necrosis and recurrence of disease after radiation therapy vis-à-vis the conventional cross-sectional imaging.

PET CLINICS

SERIES OF RELATED INTEREST

MRI Clinics of North America
Available at: MRI.theclinics.com
Neuroimaging Clinics of North America
Available at: Neuroimaging.theclinics.com
Radiologic Clinics of North America
Available at: Radiologic.theclinics.com

THE CLINICS ARE AVAILABLE ONLINE!
Access your subscription at:
www.theclinics.com

PROGRAM OBJECTIVE
The goal of the *PET Clinics* is to keep practicing radiologists and radiology residents up to date with current clinical practice in positron emission tomography by providing timely articles reviewing the state of the art in patient care.

TARGET AUDIENCE
Practicing radiologists, radiology residents, and other health care professionals who provide patient care utilizing radiologic findings.

LEARNING OBJECTIVES
Upon completion of this activity, participants will be able to:
1. Review the use of FDG PET/CT for computing baseline tumour burden before treatment, and for visualizing treatment response to immunotherapy.
2. Discuss the role of PET in assessing lung inflammatory changes induced by radiation therapy, as well as in the detection of radiation-induced cardiovascular toxicity.
3. Recognize the role of PET in radiation oncology during diagnosis and treatment of solid malignancies.

ACCREDITATION
The Elsevier Office of Continuing Medical Education (EOCME) is accredited by the Accreditation Council for Continuing Medical Education (ACCME) to provide continuing medical education for physicians.

The EOCME designates this journal-based CME activity for a maximum of 10 *AMA PRA Category 1 Credit*(s)™. Physicians should claim only the credit commensurate with the extent of their participation in the activity.

All other health care professionals requesting continuing education credit for this enduring material will be issued a certificate of participation.

DISCLOSURE OF CONFLICTS OF INTEREST
The EOCME assesses conflict of interest with its instructors, faculty, planners, and other individuals who are in a position to control the content of CME activities. All relevant conflicts of interest that are identified are thoroughly vetted by EOCME for fair balance, scientific objectivity, and patient care recommendations. EOCME is committed to providing its learners with CME activities that promote improvements or quality in healthcare and not a specific proprietary business or a commercial interest.

The planning committee, staff, authors and editors listed below have identified no financial relationships or relationships to products or devices they or their spouse/life partner have with commercial interest related to the content of this CME activity:
Erik H.J.G. Aarntzen, MD, PhD; Tony Abraham, DO, MPA; Nicolas Aide, MD, PhD; Abass Alavi, MD, MD (Hon), PhD (Hon), DSc (Hon); Sandip Basu, MBBS (Hons), DRM, Diplomate N.B., MNAMS; N. Patrik Brodin, PhD; Jason W. Chan, MD; Alexandra D. Dreyfuss, BS; Chunxiao Guo, MD; Sandra Heskamp, MD, PhD; Nicole A. Hohenstein, BA; Amir Iravani, MD, FRACP; Pegah Jahangiri, MD; Adeel Kaiser, MD; Alison Kemp; Antony Koroulakis, MD; Egesta Lopci, MD, PhD; Michel Meignan, MD, PhD; Hari Menon, BS; Jason K. Molitoris, MD, PhD; Rahul V. Parghane, MBBS, MD; Berber Piet, MD; Kevin Prigent, MD, MS; Stephanie R. Rice, MD; Shahneen Sandhu, MBBS, FRACP; Ankur M. Sharma, MD; Osman M. Siddiqui, MD; Charles B. Simone, II, MD; Peggy Tahir, MA, MLIS; Michel M. van den Heuvel, MD, PhD; Carla M. L. van Herpen, MD, PhD; John Vassallo; Vignesh Viswanathan; Sarah R. Verhoeff, MD; Vivek Verma, MD; Susan Y. Wu, MD; Sue S. Yom, MD, PhD, MAS.

The planning committee, staff, authors and editors listed below have identified financial relationships or relationships to products or devices they or their spouse/life partner have with commercial interest related to the content of this CME activity:
Michael Chuong, MD: participates in speakers bureau with Accuray Incorporated and Sirtex Medical Inc.; receives research support from AstraZeneca; participates in speakers bureau, is a consultant/advisor and receives research support from Viewray Technologies, Inc.

Rodney J. Hicks, MD, FRACP: owns stock in Telix Pharmaceuticals Limited.

Nitin Ohri, MD: consultant/advisor for and receives research support from Merck Sharp & Dohme Corp.; consultant/advisor for AstraZeneca.

Wolfgang A. Tomé, PhD: consultant/advisor for and owns stock in Archeus Technologies, Inc.; holds patents with WARF; receives research support from Accuray Incorporated, Chrysalis BioTherapeutics, Inc, and Varian Medical Systems, Inc.

UNAPPROVED/OFF-LABEL USE DISCLOSURE
The EOCME requires CME faculty to disclose to the participants:
1. When products or procedures being discussed are off-label, unlabelled, experimental, and/or investigational (not US Food and Drug Administration [FDA] approved); and
2. Any limitations on the information presented, such as data that are preliminary or that represent ongoing research, interim analyses, and/or unsupported opinions. Faculty may discuss information about pharmaceutical agents that is outside of

FDA-approved labelling. This information is intended solely for CME and is not intended to promote off-label use of these medications. If you have any questions, contact the medical affairs department of the manufacturer for the most recent prescribing information.

TO ENROLL

To enroll in the *PET Clinics* Continuing Medical Education program, call customer service at 1-800-654-2452 or sign up online at http://www.theclinics.com/home/cme. The CME program is available to subscribers for an additional annual fee of USD $235.

METHOD OF PARTICIPATION

In order to claim credit, participants must complete the following:
1. Complete enrolment as indicated above.
2. Read the activity.
3. Complete the CME Test and Evaluation. Participants must achieve a score of 70% on the test. All CME Tests and Evaluations must be completed online.

CME INQUIRIES/SPECIAL NEEDS

For all CME inquiries or special needs, please contact elsevierCME@elsevier.com

Preface
PET Imaging for Immunotherapy and Radiation Therapy

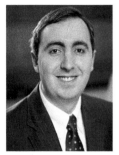 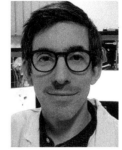 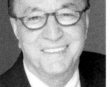

Charles B. Simone II, MD   Nicolas Aide, MD, PhD   Abass Alavi, MD

Editors

This focused issue of *PET Clinics* covers 2 important and hot topics in oncology: the use of PET imaging in assessing the efficacy of immunotherapy and the use of PET imaging in radiation oncology clinical practice.

The first part of this special issue is dedicated to immunotherapy, which has fundamentally changed the landscape of treatment for solid tumors,[1–4] although many challenges persist, such as providing prognostic information for patients, selecting patients for treatment, differentiating pseudoprogression from real progression, and identifying hyperprogression and immune-related side effects. Emerging data support the usefulness PET with fludeoxyglucose (FDG)/computed tomography (CT) for computing baseline tumor burden before treatment, and for visualizing treatment response to immunotherapy, signs of immune activation, and immune-related side effects.

The article from Prigent and colleagues provides recommendations for performing FDG-PET scanning, assessing tumor response, and reporting immune-related side effects, with representative clinical cases. A review from Hicks and colleagues details the latest evidence regarding the use of FDG-PET/CT in therapeutic monitoring of immune checkpoint inhibitors in solid tumors. Both of these articles are also meant to provide insights on the biological basis of checkpoint inhibitors used alone or in combination with other agents or radiotherapy. Also detailed is the implementation of adapted criteria for therapy monitoring in lymphoma patients, in whom FDG PET is widely used. Finally, Heskamp and colleagues review specific molecular imaging agents that can noninvasively assess global expression of immune targets.

The second part of this special issue is dedicated to the use of PET in radiation oncology, one of the primary pillars of treatment for solid malignancies. PET has increasingly well-established roles in radiation oncology for the identification of tumor to establish an initial diagnosis, to evaluate the extent of disease and clinical staging, to assess prognosis, to monitor treatment response, and to evaluate for and detect tumor recurrence following radiotherapy.[5] Furthermore, with the increasing use of advanced radiation therapy treatment techniques, including intensity-modulated radiation therapy, stereotactic body radiation therapy, and proton therapy, treatments have become more conformal and precise. As such, the need to optimally differentiate tumor from normal tissues is more important than ever, and this is a major use of PET imaging for radiation oncologists.[6]

The article by Menon and colleagues details how PET can aid in and offer considerable advantages for target volume delineation in radiation oncology. This can allow for better differentiation of tumor from normal tissues and can also better facilitate radiation dose escalation, adaptive treatment planning, and treatment optimization by risk status. Brodin and colleagues then detail the

PET Clin 15 (2020) xiii–xiv
https://doi.org/10.1016/j.cpet.2019.10.001
1556-8598/20/© 2019 Published by Elsevier Inc.

recent advancements in the role of PET for patients with locally advanced non–small cell lung cancer treated with definitive radiotherapy, for which PET can enhance prognostication of treatment outcomes, determine the definition of target volumes, and inform radiation dose modifications. Hohenstein and colleagues next focus on the ability of PET imaging to improve diagnosis, staging, radiation treatment response assessment, and outcome prognostication for patients with head and neck cancers. In the next major radiation oncology disease addressed, Rice and colleagues detail the utility of PET imaging for radiation oncology treatment planning, posttreatment surveillance, and prognosis prediction in patients with a variety of gastrointestinal malignancies, including esophageal, gastric, hepatobiliary, pancreatic, colorectal, and anal cancers.

The final 2 articles of this focused issue address emerging roles of PET in radiation oncology practice. Dreyfuss and colleagues discuss novel quantitative PET techniques that can detect radiation-induced complications. The authors focus on pulmonary and cardiac toxicities from radiotherapy, which can be associated with significant morbidity and even risks of treatment-related mortality in patients with thoracic malignancies. Finally, Parghane and Basu bridge the 2 concentrations of this focused issue together by reviewing how PET can be used to assess treatment response for both immunotherapy and radiation therapy, and they also discuss the role of more novel quantitative PET metrics, including whole-body metabolic burden, metabolic tumor volume, and total lesion glycolysis.

The intersection of immunotherapy in combination with radiation therapy is the next hot field in oncology care.[7–10] This focused issue connects both immunotherapy and radiation therapy through the dependence of each of these modalities on PET imaging.

Charles B. Simone II, MD
Department of Radiation Oncology
New York Proton Center
225 East 126th Street
New York, NY 10035, USA

Nicolas Aide, MD, PhD
Service de Médecine Nucléaire
CHU de CAEN, Avenue Côte de Nacre
Caen 1400, France

University of Normandy
Esplanade de la Paix CS 14032
Caen Cedex 5 14032, France

Abass Alavi, MD
Department of Radiology
Hospital of the University of Pennsylvania
University of Pennsylvania
3400 Spruce Street
Philadelphia, PA 19104, USA

E-mail addresses:
csimone@nyproton.com (C.B. Simone)
aide-n@chu-caen.fr (N. Aide)
Abass.Alavi@pennmedicine.upenn.edu (A. Alavi)

REFERENCES

1. Ferris RL. Immunology and immunotherapy of head and neck cancer. J Clin Oncol 2015;33(29):3293–304.
2. Sampson JH, Maus MV, June CH. Immunotherapy for brain tumors. J Clin Oncol 2017;35(21):2450–6.
3. Hirsch FR, Scagliotti GV, Mulshine JL, et al. Lung cancer: current therapies and new targeted treatments. Lancet 2017;389(10066):299–311.
4. Esteva FJ, Hubbard-Lucey VM, Tang J, et al. Immunotherapy and targeted therapy combinations in metastatic breast cancer. Lancet Oncol 2019;20(3):e175–86.
5. Simone CB 2nd, Houshmand S, Kalbasi A, et al. PET-based thoracic radiation oncology. PET Clin 2016;11(3):319–32.
6. Verma V, Choi JI, Sawant A, et al. Use of PET and other functional imaging to guide target delineation in radiation oncology. Semin Radiat Oncol 2018;28(3):171–7.
7. Simone CB 2nd, Burri SH, Heinzerling JH. Novel radiotherapy approaches for lung cancer: combining radiation therapy with targeted and immunotherapies. Transl Lung Cancer Res 2015;4(5):545–52.
8. Bauml JM, Mick R, Ciunci C, et al. Pembrolizumab after completion of locally ablative therapy for oligometastatic non-small cell lung cancer: a phase 2 trial. JAMA Oncol 2019;5(9):1283–90.
9. Badiyan SN, Roach MC, Chuong MD, et al. Combining immunotherapy with radiation therapy in thoracic oncology. J Thorac Dis 2018;10(suppl 21):S2492–507.
10. Pitroda SP, Chmura SJ, Weichselbaum RR. Integration of radiotherapy and immunotherapy for treatment of oligometastases. Lancet Oncol 2019;20(8):e434–42.

¹⁸F-Fludeoxyglucose PET/Computed Tomography for Assessing Tumor Response to Immunotherapy and Detecting Immune-Related Side Effects
A Checklist for the PET Reader

Kevin Prigent, MD, MS[a,b], Nicolas Aide, MD, PhD[b,c],*

KEYWORDS

- FDG • PET • Immunotherapy • Immune-related side effects • Pseudoprogression
- Hyperprogression • Therapy monitoring

KEY POINTS

- ¹⁸F-Fludeoxyglucose PET is the only imaging modality capable of visualizing treatment response to immunotherapy, signs of immune activation (spleen uptake and so forth), and immune-related side effects.
- Because it is known that patients experiencing immune-relate side effects are more likely to respond to treatment, discriminating between pseudoprogression and real progression and identification of hyperprogression is key for patient care.
- Conventional PET criteria (European Organization for Research and Treatment of Cancer and PET Evaluation Response Criteria In Solid Tumours) can overlook pseudoprogression, leading to the use of immune-modified PET criteria.

BACKGROUND
Immune Checkpoint Inhibitors

Immunotherapy, which radically differs from other strategies in relying on the reactivation of the immune system to recognize and kill cancer cells, has recently emerged as an important advance in cancer treatment.[1] The use of immunomodulatory monoclonal antibodies that directly enhance the function of components of the antitumor immune response, such as T cells, or block immunologic checkpoints that would otherwise restrain effective anti-tumor immunity, has recently been actively investigated in oncology.

To date, the main immunotherapeutic approach that has been translated into survival benefit and is currently used in practice is the blockade of immune checkpoints. Broadly, the 2 most effective classes of agent are directed, alone or in combination, toward cytotoxic T lymphocyte-associated protein 4 (CTLA-4) or the programmed cell death protein 1 (PD1) or the PD1/programmed cell death protein ligand 1 (PD1/PD-L1) axis, which are negative regulators of T-cell immune function.[2]

The CTLA-4 inhibitor, ipilimumab, has been shown to improve survival rates in melanoma patients. PD1/PD-L1 inhibitors (of which the first

Disclosure Statement: The authors have nothing to disclose.
[a] Nuclear Medicine Department, University Hospital, Caen, France; [b] Service de Médecine Nucléaire, CHU de CAEN, Avenue Côte de Nacre, Caen, France; [c] University of Normandy, France
* Corresponding author. Service de Médecine Nucléaire, CHU de CAEN, Avenue Côte de Nacre, Caen, France.
E-mail address: nicolasaide0@gmail.com

https://doi.org/10.1016/j.cpet.2019.08.006

pet.theclinics.com

validated agents were pembrolizumab and nivolu-mab) have been shown to improve survival rates among patients with various tumor types, including melanoma, lung, head and neck, and bladder can-cers. Typically, these drugs are given intravenously every 2 to 3 weeks, and a durable complete response has been observed in a variable but small proportion of patients. Patients whose tumors or immune cells express PD-L1 have a higher likeli-hood of benefiting from treatment with PD1/PD-L1 inhibitors, although PD-L1-negative patients have also been shown to respond.

Because not all patients respond to single-agent immunotherapy, hundreds of combination trials are ongoing. At the time of the writing of this article, more than 2916 trials using immunotherapy are listing on clinicaltrial.gov. Among these trials, 23 use ^{18}F-Fludeoxyglucose (FDG) PET as a tool for therapy monitoring. Different combination stra-tegies are under investigation, including with stan-dard chemotherapy, targeted agents, and antiangiogenic agents. Because radiation induces the release of tumor antigens, also known as neo-antigens, there is strong rationale supporting the use of combinations of external and immune checkpoint inhibitors, with patients benefiting from the so-called abscopal effect.[3]

Immune-Related Side Effects

By reactivating the immune system, these immu-notherapies have led to the development of new toxicity profiles, also called immune-related adverse events (irAE). IrAEs can involve many or-gan systems, and their management is radically different from that of adverse events from cyto-toxic drugs.[4] There is a wide variety of irAEs, with the endocrine, lung, cutaneous, and gastroin-testinal systems being the most commonly affected. The irAE pattern is different across im-mune checkpoint inhibitor classes and could be driven by the different patterns of immune cell acti-vation that can occur with different classes of im-mune therapy.[5] The rapid identification of these irAEs and treatment with corticoids[6,7] can improve patient outcomes, without reduction in treatment efficacy.[8,9]

Other details on available inhibitors, their bio-logic rationale, and irAE can be found elsewhere.[10–16]

Pseudoprogression and Hyperprogression

Different patterns of response to immunothera-peutic agents were also observed from those to chemotherapeutic and molecularly targeted agents. First, responses usually occur early, but can also be delayed. Second, responses may be preceded by apparent disease progression, defined as pseudoprogression. These patterns of response were mainly initially reported in patients with melanoma receiving anti-CLTA4 agents, with approximately 15% of patients experiencing pseudoprogression,[17] and led to adapted morphologic criteria on computed tomography (CT), namely the irRECIST criteria.[17–19] Tumors other than melanoma show lower cases of pseu-doprogression (<3%), especially with the use of anti-PD1/PD-L1 agents.

More recently, hyperprogression was described as an acceleration of tumor growth kinetics.[20,21] Indeed, some phase 3 trials have illustrated worse overall survival rates in patients receiving immune checkpoint inhibitors than in control patients dur-ing the first few months, supporting the concept of hyperprogression.[19,22] Although these studies had no control arm, they suggested that immuno-therapy might be detrimental in some patients with cancer.[20,21,23]

^{18}F-Fludeoxyglucose PET for Immunotherapy Response Assessment: Evolution of Metabolic Response Criteria

The first PET-based response criteria were pro-posed by the European Organization for Research and Treatment of Cancer (EORTC) in 1999,[24] and The PET Evaluation Response Criteria In Solid Tu-mours (PERCIST) were later published in 2009.[25,26] PERCIST are rather similar to the EORTC criteria, and these criteria often produce very similar results, with agreement reported to range between 0.76 and 1.[27] Whereas EORTC is based on the use of maximum standardized up-take value (SUV_{max}), PERCIST recommend SUV lean (SUV normalized by lean body mass, or SUL) for the assessment of tumor response and the identification of a minimum tumor SUL equiva-lent to 1.5 times the mean SUL of the liver for a lesion to be selected as target lesion. PERCIST also recommend the measurement of SUL in up to 5 tumors (up to 2 per organ). The latter were also the first criteria using SUL_{peak}, which can be measured within a 1-cm^3 spherical volume of in-terest (VOI).

The EORTC criteria do not specify the number of lesions to be measured or the minimum measur-able lesion uptake, whereas PERCIST have re-quirements regarding target selection (typically the hottest lesions, from 1 to 5 and no more than 2 per organ). For PERCIST criteria, the measurable target lesion is the single most intense tumor site on pretreatment and posttreatment scans, which means that the target lesion may receive different pretreatment and posttreatment.

Based on the SUL_{peak} and SUV_{max} variation between the pretreatment and posttreatment scans, patients were classified according to PERCIST and EORTC as follows:

- *Complete metabolic response*: complete resolution of ^{18}F-FDG uptake in the tumor volume, with tumor SUL lower than liver SUL and background blood pool, and disappearance of all lesions if multiple.
- *Partial metabolic response*: at least 30% (PERCIST) or 25% (EORTC) reduction in tumor uptake.
- *Stable metabolic disease*: less than 30% (PERCIST) or 25% (EORTC) increase, or less than 30% or 25% (EORTC) decrease in tumor ^{18}F-FDG SUL_{peak} and no new lesions.
- *Progressive metabolic disease* (PMD): greater than 30% (PERCIST) or 25% (EORTC) increase in ^{18}F-FDG tumor SUL_{peak} within the tumor or appearance of new lesions.

Because of the change of patient classification after the appearance of a new lesion as PMD for both EORTC and PERCIST, these criteria would be misled in the case of pseudoprogression. Indeed, the EORTC criteria were the first to be applied for the assessment of response of solid tumors to immunotherapy. In that first report, the investigators recognized the appearance of new lesions, conventionally defining disease progression as being a potential cause of response misclassification that occurred in 4 out of 22 melanoma patients scanned after 2 cycles of Ipilimumab.[28]

Within the last few years, several modified PET evaluation criteria have been proposed, mainly in series of melanoma patients receiving Ipilimumab.[28–32] This article does not aim to describe these studies in detail; they can be found in the recent report of the European Association of Nuclear Medicine on immunotherapy assessment.

To briefly summarize, efforts tended to better evaluate the whole tumor burden and not be misled by the appearance of new lesions wrongly classifying patients experiencing pseudoprogression as PMD. Most of the published series included a limited number of patients and focused on melanoma patients receiving ipililumab.

PERCIST were the most heavily studied criteria, because they recommend to select up to 5 (hottest) lesions, which can be adapted to search for new lesions deemed to be pseudoprogressive. Several investigators also advised an early follow-up study to confirm or exclude pseudoprogression.

RECOMMENDATION ON PET SCANNING AND REPORTING
PET Protocol

First, it is important to remember patients should be scanned on the same PET system for baseline and posttreatment scans, because it is known that reconstruction inconsistencies may strongly alter EORTC and PERCIST classification. This issue would obviously also apply to modified PERCIST criteria.

Apart from the usual compliance to PET tumor imaging guidelines and harmonizing standards, several points regarding the PET acquisition protocol need to be raised.[33–35] First, although including the brain in the field of view is not systematic for most of the PET centers, the skull base should be included, so that immune-related side effects involving the pituitary gland are observed (**Fig. 1**A, B). Second, in patients with melanoma with a primary location in the lower limbs, a whole-body acquisition is recommended (**Fig. 1**C, D).

The number of cycles of immunotherapy since the baseline PET scan and the date of the last infusion are also given. Patients may have received several lines of immunotherapy, for example, because they experienced a toxicity requiring a first line to be withdrawn, and are rechallenged with another drug after recovery of irAEs.

When to Perform ^{18}F-Fludeoxyglucose PET?

FDG PET imaging should be performed before the start of immunotherapy. The metabolic information obtained at this time allows adequate restaging and proper evaluation of disease extent at baseline. Based on a given tumor board, the scan can be repeated at the first treatment response evaluation, which in most cancer types is 8 or 9 weeks after the start of immunotherapy (generally after 2 or 3 cycles of treatment), depending on the regimen used. It is noteworthy that some patients receiving nivolumab may receive a flat dose by injection every 4 weeks. In that case, patients receive the same total dose as for the 2-week injection period, and it can be recommended to scan them after a single injection if early therapy assessment is required. Subsequent imaging with FDG-PET is recommended regularly during treatment and at the end of immunotherapy, before treatment stops.

In the case of irAEs, which are very likely to be visualized on PET imaging, FDG PET can be used after treatment withdrawal and/or corticosteroids treatment, to check whether the side effects have been resolved and to be used as a new baseline scan before rechallenging with

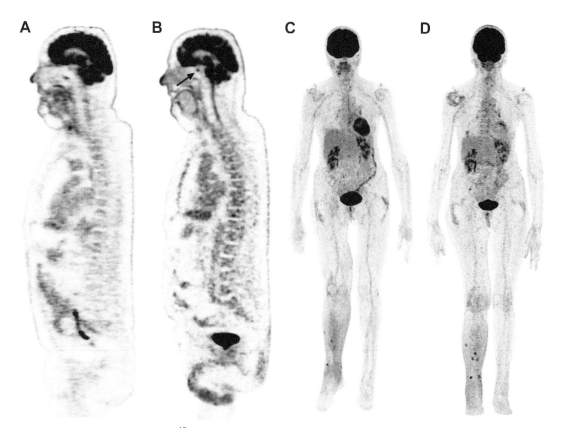

Fig. 1. PET protocol. Serial sagittal ^{18}F FDG PET and PET-CT, including the skull in different phases of the disease in a 74-year-old man affected by a metastatic melanoma of the right thigh. (*A*) Baseline before introduction of immunotherapy and (*B*) after 6 courses of nivolumab, showing a related hypermetabolism in the pituitary gland (*arrow*) owing to nivolumab toxicity in an asymptomatic patient. Serial ^{18}F FDG maximum intensity projection (MIP), including the skull and lower limbs in different phases of the disease in an 82-year-old woman affected by a melanoma of the right ankle with in transit metastases of the right lower limb and the lung. (*C*) Baseline before introduction of immunotherapy and (*D*) after 2 courses of nivolumab, showing a metabolic progression in the right lower limb and lung.

immunotherapy or the start of another line of treatment, whether it is chemotherapy or tyrosine kinase inhibitors.

How to Assess and Report Immune-Related Signs

Inflammatory reactions can occur during the treatment and are associated with high glucose consumption, which may be associated with pseudoprogression and irAEs and can lead to misinterpretation of FDG PET images. Response assessment during immunotherapy can therefore be rather challenging. However, FDG PET can show dynamic adaptation of the immune response to checkpoint inhibitors.[36,37] Moreover, being a whole-body modality, it also allows precise localization of irAEs, which can occasionally become life-threatening; for example, colitis, pneumonitis, and pancreatitis. Furthermore, the occurrence of

irAEs and the possibility of detecting them on PET may be an additional factor predicting response to immunotherapy, given the evidence that appearance of irAEs is associated with a better response to PD1 inhibitors in patients with melanoma or NSCLC.[14,38]

Although potentially immune-related inflammatory findings on FDG PET should be reported, these will not necessarily be associated with clinical symptoms (ie, irAEs). However, clinicians should be made aware of their presence so that complementary tests and clinical monitoring can be performed, because medical intervention may be necessary in selected cases. **Fig. 2**A–C displays colitis, whereas **Fig. 2**D–F illustrates a metformin-induced pseudocolitis pattern.

The first sign of immune activity to be checked is spleen enlargement and/or increased uptake leading to an inversion of the liver-to-spleen uptake ratio (**Fig. 3**). Reactive nodes in the drainage basin of

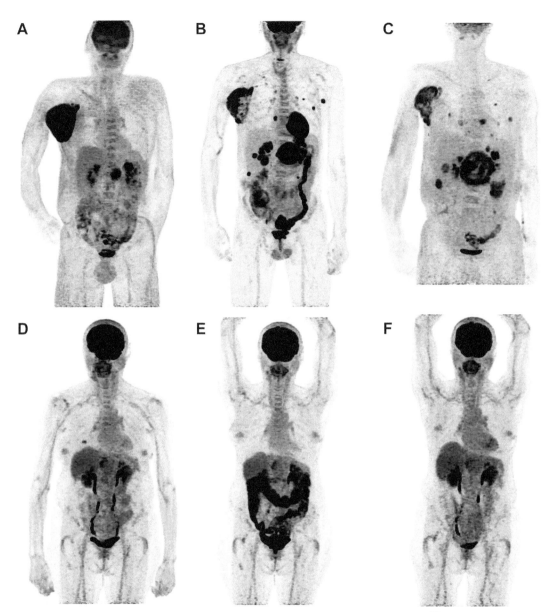

Fig. 2. Seeking immune-related side effect on FDG PET: beware of the outlier! Serial ^{18}F FDG MIP in different phases of the disease in a 65-year-old woman affected by a choroid melanoma with hepatic lymph node involvement. (*A*) PET after 6 courses of pembrolizumab, (*B*) PET after 8 courses of pembrolizumab, showing a diffuse colic hypermetabolism with diarrhea related to immunotherapy toxicity, confirmed by endoscopy-guided biopsies, leading to the withdrawal of pembrolizumab and the use of corticosteroids. (*C*) Patient was switched to nivolumab and FDG PET after 1 course of nivolumab allowed checking for the absence of any recurrence of the colitis. Serial ^{18}F FDG PET in different phases of the disease in a diabetic 59-year-old man affected by a metastatic melanoma under metformin. In most of the PET centers, withdrawal of metformin is planned to avoid intense uptake in the colon and small bowel. (*D*) PET baseline before introduction of immunotherapy with 1.34 g/L of glycemia. (*E*) PET after 2 courses of pembrolizumab, showing a diffuse colic hypermetabolism thought to be irAE colitis. However, the endoscopy was normal, and normal glycemia (0.65 g/L) at the time of the interim PET was likely due to a lack of observance of the recommended discontinuation of metformin 2 days before the FDG PET/CT. (*F*) PET after 5 courses of pembrolizumab showing the absence of colic hypermetabolism with 1.92 g/L of glycemia.

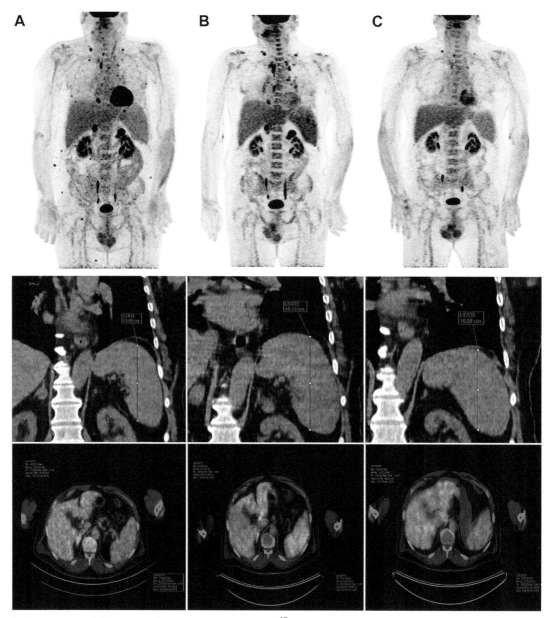

Fig. 3. How to seek immune activation on FDG PET. Serial ^{18}F FDG PET/CT in different phases of the disease in a 61-year-old man affected by a melanoma of the left forearm with subcutaneous lymph nodes and bilateral adrenal glands involvement. (*A*) Baseline PET before introduction of immunotherapy and (*B*) after 2 courses of nivolumab, showing diffuse osteomedullary hypermetabolism, an inversion of the spleen-to-liver ratio associated with an increase in the spleen dimensions in line with a lymphocyte activation. This pattern precedes (*C*), an excellent partial metabolic response that is observed after 5 courses of nivolumab in all lesions.

the primary tumor may also be seen. To date, there are no consensus guidelines on how to report spleen uptake. Also, uptake in other lymphoid organs has been reported, namely, thymus, ileocecal valve, and healthy bone marrow.[36] In their study, Seban and colleagues[39] reported the use of SUV_{max} obtained with a 2-cm VOI for the spleen and a 15-mm VOI placed at the center of the first lumbar vertebrae for bone marrow. The investigators also used a 3-cm VOI in the liver to compute spleen-to-liver ratio and bone marrow-to-liver ratio. In this way, the liver VOI may also be used for PERCIST or immune-modified PERCIST. Therefore, although reporting multiple target of immune activation is likely to be time consuming in routine practice, the authors suggest that the

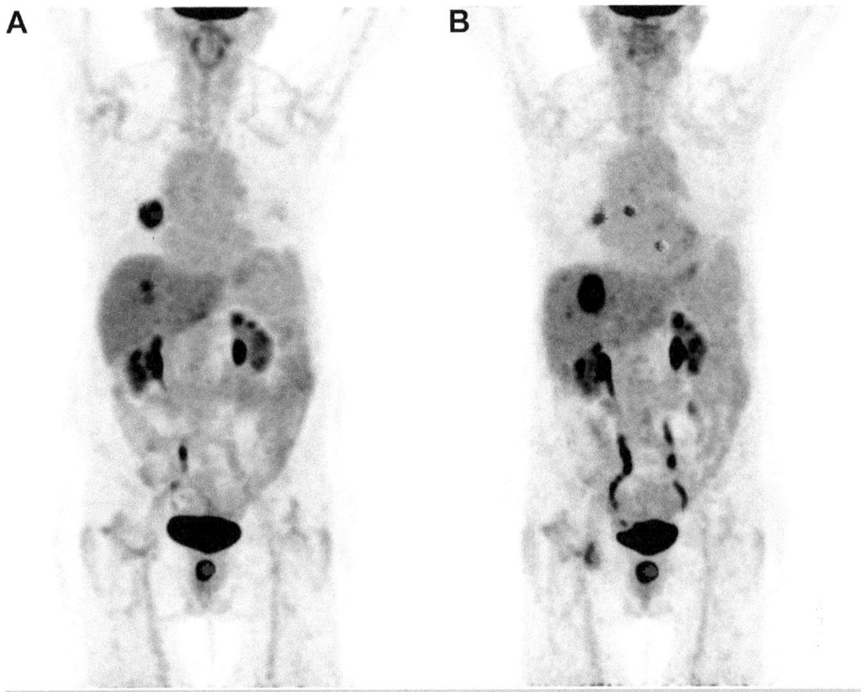

Target	Baseline EARL SUL peak		Interim EARL SUL peak	
1	15.32	Anal	17.41	Anal
2	5.59	Lung	7.77	Hepatic
3	2.85	Hepatic	2.55	Lymph Node
4	2.35	Hepatic	2.3	Lung
5	1.12	Bone	2.3	Bone
	27.23		32.33 : △ -18.72%	
PERCIST5			PMD	
imPERCIST5			SMD	

Fig. 4. Evaluating tumor response: PERCIST versus immune-adapted PERCIST. Serial ^{18}F FDG MIP in different phases of the disease in a 73-year-old woman affected by a melanoma of the anal canal with lung and lymph node hepatic metastasis. (A) PET baseline before introduction of immunotherapy and (B) after 6 courses of nivolumab, showing the appearance of new lesions. This pattern classifies the patient with PMD according to the PERCIST5 criteria, but stable metabolic disease is found when using imPERCIST5. EARL, EANM Research Ltd; SMD, stable metabolic disease.

PET reader could report SUV metrics in 2 VOIs in the liver and in the spleen at the same level and compute the liver-to-spleen ratio (see **Fig. 3**).

Because every organ can be involved by the immune infiltrate, it is important to use the baseline scan data not only to compare changes in uptake in the target lesions but also to check that intense uptake deemed to be an immune-related sign was not present on the baseline scan. On the contrary, diffuse and intense uptake in these organs is likely to be an immune-related sign.

One should also consider whether the pattern of new nodal uptake suggests sarcoidosis,

especially bilateral hilar and mediastinal uptake associated with portocaval nodal uptake.

Therapy Assessment

Depending on the availability of the SUV$_{peak}$ metric on the workstation used, either the EORTC PET response criteria or PERCIST can be used to report FDG uptake changes in target lesions. However, care should be taken when reporting PET results in patients in whom disease progression is suspected, because of the difference in patterns of response to immunotherapy from those to conventional chemotherapy and other molecularly targeted therapies, especially during the first few cycles of treatment. One should be aware of the possibility of pseudoprogression, having in mind that this should only be considered when the clinical condition of the patient is concomitantly improving. In patients whose clinical condition is not improving and who have disease progression on imaging, one should discontinue immunotherapy. The risk of continuing treatment beyond progression is that it may prevent commencement of a new line of treatment once the progression is confirmed because of clinical deterioration.

In patients with apparent disease progression, the number and location of new lesions should be reported, excluding pathologic foci in organs deemed to be due to the immune infiltrate. Indeed, a recent study suggested that the appearance of 4 or more new lesions of less than 1 cm in functional diameter or 3 or more new lesions of more than 1 cm in functional diameter is likely to be due to a real progression rather than pseudoprogression.[31]

The PET reader should be aware of the importance of interrupting treatment early if hyperprogression is suspected, because this pattern is more frequent in elderly patients.

As far as selecting which criteria should be used, several series have reported various modifications of PERCIST. However, none of them have proposed a recommended use for daily practice. However, as PERCIST have become used more and more often for the evaluation of chemotherapy and molecularly targeted therapy, the authors think that it is appropriate for the PET community to use these modified criteria, especially in the case where patients' progression is suspected based on the appearance of new suspicious lesions. In this case, it can be recommended to use imPERCIST,[40] where the 5 hottest lesions are selected and a new hot lesion would not classify the patient as PMD, unless the variation in the sum of the 5 hottest lesions between baseline and interim PET is greater than 30% (**Fig. 4**). Gathering, pooling, and analyzing that kind of data within national or international observational studies, in addition to the metrics mentioned in later discussion, would be a useful way of improving the use and the visibility of FDG PET for therapy assessment in patients receiving immunotherapy.

Perspectives

In addition to conventional SUV metrics, one could consider recording metabolic active tumor volume (MATV) and Total Lesion Glycolycis (TLG) before and after treatment,[41,42] again excluding uptake in organs deemed to be due to the immune infiltrate. Indeed, MATV could be seen as the PET counterpart of iRECIST, where the sum of all lesions is used. More recently, PET texture analysis (TF)[43,44] has emerged in the field of cancerology and has shown promising results in predicting response to treatment and as a risk stratification tool. In addition to their potential role as prognosticators, FDG PET heterogeneity parameters in differentiating between pseudoprogression and real progression could be evaluated, on the basis that pseudoprogressing lesions, because of the immune infiltrate, may harbor different TF patterns.

The recent evolution in PET images analysis based on machine learning and central neutral network could make computation of MATV and TLG easier. In particular, automatic or semiautomatic computation of tumor MATV/TLG and splenic MATV/TLG would be useful to the PET reader to assess the whole tumor burden together with signs of immune activation, while maintaining the throughput of a busy PET center.

REFERENCES

1. Lheureux S, Denoyelle C, Ohashi PS, et al. Molecularly targeted therapies in cancer: a guide for the nuclear medicine physician. Eur J Nucl Med Mol Imaging 2017;44(Suppl 1):41–54.
2. Mellman I, Coukos G, Dranoff G. Cancer immunotherapy comes of age. Nature 2011;480(7378):480–9.
3. Reynders K, Illidge T, Siva S, et al. The abscopal effect of local radiotherapy: using immunotherapy to make a rare event clinically relevant. Cancer Treat Rev 2015;41(6):503–10.
4. Cousin S, Italiano A. Molecular pathways: immune checkpoint antibodies and their toxicities. Clin Cancer Res 2016;22(18):4550–5.
5. Khoja L, Day D, Wei-Wu Chen T, et al. Tumour- and class-specific patterns of immune-related adverse events of immune checkpoint inhibitors: a systematic review. Ann Oncol 2017;28(10):2377–85.
6. Fujii T, Colen RR, Bilen MA, et al. Incidence of immune-related adverse events and its association with treatment outcomes: the MD Anderson Cancer Center experience. Invest New Drugs 2018;36(4):638–46.
7. Geukes Foppen MH, Rozeman EA, van Wilpe S, et al. Immune checkpoint inhibition-related colitis: symptoms, endoscopic features, histology and response to management. ESMO Open 2018;3(1):e000278.
8. Harmankaya K, Erasim C, Koelblinger C, et al. Continuous systemic corticosteroids do not affect the ongoing regression of metastatic melanoma for more than two years following ipilimumab therapy. Med Oncol 2011;28(4):1140–4.

9. Weber JS, Hodi FS, Wolchok JD, et al. Safety profile of nivolumab monotherapy: a pooled analysis of patients with advanced melanoma. J Clin Oncol 2017; 35(7):785–92.

10. Pardoll DM. The blockade of immune checkpoints in cancer immunotherapy. Nat Rev Cancer 2012;12(4): 252–64.

11. Merelli B, Massi D, Cattaneo L, et al. Targeting the PD1/PD-L1 axis in melanoma: biological rationale, clinical challenges and opportunities. Crit Rev Oncol Hematol 2014;89(1):140–65.

12. Bardhan K, Anagnostou T, Boussiotis VA. The PD1: PD-L1/2 pathway from discovery to clinical implementation. Front Immunol 2016;7:550.

13. Buchbinder EI, Desai A. CTLA-4 and PD-1 pathways: similarities, differences, and implications of their inhibition. Am J Clin Oncol 2016;39(1):98–106.

14. Friedman CF, Proverbs-Singh TA, Postow MA. Treatment of the immune-related adverse effects of immune checkpoint inhibitors: a review. JAMA Oncol 2016;2(10):1346–53.

15. Spain L, Diem S, Larkin J. Management of toxicities of immune checkpoint inhibitors. Cancer Treat Rev 2016;44:51–60.

16. Martins F, Sofiya L, Sykiotis GP, et al. Adverse effects of immune-checkpoint inhibitors: epidemiology, management and surveillance. Nat Rev Clin Oncol 2019;16(9):563–80.

17. Wolchok JD, Hoos A, O'Day S, et al. Guidelines for the evaluation of immune therapy activity in solid tumors: immune-related response criteria. Clin Cancer Res 2009;15(23):7412–20.

18. Nishino M, Giobbie-Hurder A, Gargano M, et al. Developing a common language for tumor response to immunotherapy: immune-related response criteria using unidimensional measurements. Clin Cancer Res 2013;19(14):3936–43.

19. Hodi FS, Hwu WJ, Kefford R, et al. Evaluation of immune-related response criteria and RECIST v1.1 in patients with advanced melanoma treated with pembrolizumab. J Clin Oncol 2016;34(13):1510–7.

20. Champiat S, Dercle L, Ammari S, et al. Hyperprogressive disease is a new pattern of progression in cancer patients treated by anti-PD-1/PD-L1. Clin Cancer Res 2017;23(8):1920–8.

21. Saada-Bouzid E, Defaucheux C, Karabajakian A, et al. Hyperprogression during anti-PD-1/PD-L1 therapy in patients with recurrent and/or metastatic head and neck squamous cell carcinoma. Ann Oncol 2017;28(7):1605–11.

22. Ferris RL, Blumenschein G Jr, Fayette J, et al. Nivolumab for recurrent squamous-cell carcinoma of the head and neck. N Engl J Med 2016;375(19): 1856–67.

23. Sharon E. Can an immune checkpoint inhibitor (sometimes) make things worse? Clin Cancer Res 2017;23(8):1879–81.

24. Young H, Baum R, Cremerius U, et al. Measurement of clinical and subclinical tumour response using [18F]-fluorodeoxyglucose and positron emission tomography: review and 1999 EORTC recommendations. European Organization for Research and Treatment of Cancer (EORTC) PET Study Group. Eur J Cancer 1999;35(13):1773–82.

25. Wahl RL, Jacene H, Kasamon Y, et al. From RECIST to PERCIST: evolving considerations for PET response criteria in solid tumors. J Nucl Med 2009; 50(Suppl 1):122s–50s.

26. O JH, Wahl RL. PERCIST in perspective. Nucl Med Mol Imaging 2018;52(1):1–4.

27. Pinker K, Riedl C, Weber WA. Evaluating tumor response with FDG PET: updates on PERCIST, comparison with EORTC criteria and clues to future developments. Eur J Nucl Med Mol Imaging 2017; 44(Suppl 1):55–66.

28. Sachpekidis C, Larribere L, Pan L, et al. Predictive value of early 18F-FDG PET/CT studies for treatment response evaluation to ipilimumab in metastatic melanoma: preliminary results of an ongoing study. Eur J Nucl Med Mol Imaging 2015;42(3):386–96.

29. Breki CM, Dimitrakopoulou-Strauss A, Hassel J, et al. Fractal and multifractal analysis of PET/CT images of metastatic melanoma before and after treatment with ipilimumab. EJNMMI Res 2016;6(1):61.

30. Cho SY, Lipson EJ, Im HJ, et al. Prediction of response to immune checkpoint inhibitor therapy using early-time-point (18)F-FDG PET/CT imaging in patients with advanced melanoma. J Nucl Med 2017;58(9):1421–8.

31. Anwar H, Sachpekidis C, Winkler J, et al. Absolute number of new lesions on (18)F-FDG PET/CT is more predictive of clinical response than SUV changes in metastatic melanoma patients receiving ipilimumab. Eur J Nucl Med Mol Imaging 2018; 45(3):376–83.

32. Sachpekidis C, Anwar H, Winkler J, et al. The role of interim (18)F-FDG PET/CT in prediction of response to ipilimumab treatment in metastatic melanoma. Eur J Nucl Med Mol Imaging 2018;45(8):1289–96.

33. Boellaard R, Delgado-Bolton R, Oyen WJ, et al. FDG PET/CT: EANM procedure guidelines for tumour imaging: version 2.0. Eur J Nucl Med Mol Imaging 2015;42(2):328–54.

34. Aide N, Lasnon C, Veit-Haibach P, et al. EANM/EARL harmonization strategies in PET quantification: from daily practice to multicentre oncological studies. Eur J Nucl Med Mol Imaging 2017;44(Suppl 1): 17–31.

35. Lasnon C, Enilorac B, Popotte H, et al. Impact of the EARL harmonization program on automatic delineation of metabolic active tumour volumes (MATVs). EJNMMI Res 2017;7(1):30.

36. Tsai KK, Pampaloni MH, Hope C, et al. Increased FDG avidity in lymphoid tissue associated with

response to combined immune checkpoint blockade. J Immunother Cancer 2016;4:58.

37. Wachsmann JW, Ganti R, Peng F. Immune-mediated disease in ipilimumab immunotherapy of melanoma with FDG PET-CT. Acad Radiol 2017;24(1):111–5.

38. Haratani K, Hayashi H, Chiba Y, et al. Association of immune-related adverse events with nivolumab efficacy in non-small-cell lung cancer. JAMA Oncol 2018;4(3):374–8.

39. Seban RD, Nemer JS, Marabelle A, et al. Prognostic and theranostic 18F-FDG PET biomarkers for anti-PD1 immunotherapy in metastatic melanoma: association with outcome and transcriptomics. Eur J Nucl Med Mol Imaging 2019;46(11):2298–310.

40. Ito K, Teng R, Schoder H, et al. 18)F-FDG PET/CT for monitoring of ipilimumab therapy in patients with metastatic melanoma. J Nucl Med 2019;60(3):335–41.

41. Kong BY, Menzies AM, Saunders CA, et al. Residual FDG-PET metabolic activity in metastatic melanoma patients with prolonged response to anti-PD-1 therapy. Pigment Cell Melanoma Res 2016;29(5):572–7.

42. Kaira K, Higuchi T, Naruse I, et al. Metabolic activity by (18)F-FDG-PET/CT is predictive of early response after nivolumab in previously treated NSCLC. Eur J Nucl Med Mol Imaging 2018;45(1):56–66.

43. Chicklore S, Goh V, Siddique M, et al. Quantifying tumour heterogeneity in 18F-FDG PET/CT imaging by texture analysis. Eur J Nucl Med Mol Imaging 2013;40(1):133–40.

44. Lasnon C, Majdoub M, Lavigne B, et al. 18)F-FDG PET/CT heterogeneity quantification through textural features in the era of harmonisation programs: a focus on lung cancer. Eur J Nucl Med Mol Imaging 2016;43(13):2324–35.

^{18}F-fluorodeoxyglucose Positron Emission Tomography/Computed Tomography for Assessing Tumor Response to Immunotherapy in Solid Tumors
Melanoma and Beyond

Rodney J. Hicks, MD, FRACP[a,b,*], Amir Iravani, MD, FRACP[a,b], Shahneen Sandhu, MBBS, FRACP[a,c]

KEYWORDS

- FDG • PET/CT • Immunotherapy • Therapeutic monitoring • Melanoma
- Non-small cell lung cancer • Biomarkers

KEY POINTS

- Recent development of immune check-point inhibitors has fundamentally changed the landscape of treatment for several diseases that previously had a dismal prognosis and no effective therapies.
- The complexity of the immune response and the diversity of targets challenges conventional conceptual frameworks used in selecting and monitoring treatment.
- Imaging and tissue biomarkers are being actively sought but are constrained by the biological, spatial, and temporal heterogeneity of the processes involved.
- As yet, there are few studies that provide clarity on how to interpret ^{18}F-fluorodeoxyglucose Positron Emission Tomography/Computed Tomography in the context of therapeutic monitoring of immune check-point inhibitors.
- Patterns of response are becoming apparent and combined with ability to detect immune-related inflammatory changes suggest that ^{18}F-fluorodeoxyglucose Positron Emission Tomography/Computed Tomography will provide useful clinical guidance early during therapy.

INTRODUCTION

Although the role of the immune system in modulating the behavior of cancers has long been suspected and the focus of prior therapeutic interventions, the recent development of immune check-point inhibitors (ICIs) has fundamentally changed the landscape of treatment for solid

Disclosure Statement: Professor Hicks is supported by a Practitioner Fellowship of the National Health and Medical Research Council of Australia (APP1108050). He holds shares in Telix Pharmaceuticals. The other authors have nothing to disclose.

[a] Sir Peter MacCallum Department of Oncology, The University of Melbourne, Australia; [b] Cancer Imaging, The Peter MacCallum Cancer Centre, Melbourne, Australia; [c] Department of Medical Oncology, the Peter MacCallum Cancer Centre, Melbourne, Australia
* Corresponding author. Peter MacCallum Cancer Centre, Locked Bag 1 A'Beckett St, Melbourne, Victoria 8006, Australia.
E-mail address: rod.hicks@petermac.org

PET Clin 15 (2020) 11–22
https://doi.org/10.1016/j.cpet.2019.08.007

tumors that previously had a dismal prognosis and no effective therapies. These include advanced melanoma and lung cancer as well as cancers with mismatch repair defects. The complexity of the immune response and the diversity of targets challenges conventional conceptual frameworks used in selecting and monitoring treatment, especially because these agents are increasingly being combined with other cancer therapies. Imaging and tissue biomarkers are being actively sought but are constrained by the biological, spatial, and temporal heterogeneity of the processes involved. The limitations of anatomic imaging in assessing response to ICIs have been recognized by the adaptation of the Response Evaluation Criteria in Solid Tumors (RECIST) to incorporate new rules by which to deal with the potential for apparent progression that subsequently resolves, which has been called pseudoprogression. Although the assessment of glycolytic metabolism using ^{18}F-fluorodeoxyglucose Positron Emission Tomography/Computed Tomography (FDG PET/CT) has generally served us well in the monitoring of response to chemotherapy and radiotherapy, it has become increasingly apparent that the uptake of FDG in tumor is much more complex than simply reflecting glucose use by cancer cells and the number and viability of those cells after treatment. The tumor microenvironment (TME) as well as metabolic signals from stromal and immune cells contribute to apparent uptake of FDG and changes in the contribution of these factors to the intensity and pattern of uptake may vary between classes of ICIs and in different cancers. As yet, there are relatively few studies that provide clarity on how these disparate responses impact FDG PET/CT and its interpretation in the context of therapeutic monitoring. This review details the latest evidence regarding the use of FDG PET/CT in therapeutic monitoring of ICIs.

THE ERA OF IMMUNE CHECK-POINT INHIBITORS

The importance of ICIs to the management of cancer was recognized by the 2018 Nobel Prize in Physiology or Medicine for discovery of key negative regulators (check-points) of the immune system; cytotoxic T-lymphocyte-associated antigen (CTLA)-4 and programmed death (PD)-1, leading to the development of anti–CTLA-4 (ipilumumab)[1] and anti–PD-1 (pembrolizumab)[2] monoclonal antibodies as the first generation of ICIs. These agents have been supplemented by several other ICIs directed against PD-1 (nivolumab) and its ligand, PD ligand (PD-L)1 (atezolizumab, durvalumab, and avelumab). These agents have all been

approved for clinical use in various cancer settings and several ICIs are in clinical trial evaluation. Although ICIs yield responses in a minority of patients, dramatic and, most impressively, durable remissions of disease can occur in previously invariably, and often rapidly, fatal cancers. For example, in a series of 270 patients with metastatic melanoma, renal cell carcinoma, and non–small cell lung cancer (NSCLC), 5-year survival rates were 34%, 28%, and 16%, respectively.[3] In the hope of further improving response rates, while leveraging the duration of response seen with ICIs, a large number of combination ICIs strategies with standard and novel treatments are being developed for possible therapeutic synergy.[4] These include targeted therapy[5] and chemotherapy that are intended to alter the TME or make the tumor more immunogenic by varied mechanisms including increased major histocompatibility complex class I expression, improved tumor antigen presentation, and cross-priming of cytotoxic T lymphocytes with the goal of increasing immune infiltrates or decreasing immunosuppressive cytokines.[6] The possibility of inducing immunogenic cell death by using radiation is one such approach. This is currently being widely evaluated with the goal of invoking responses in remote, nonirradiated sites through so-called abscopal effects.[7] It has also been argued that irradiating more sites might increase efficacy through wider presentation of tumor-associated antigens (TAAs).[8] This approach may also be of relevance to the combination of radionuclide therapy with immunotherapy, particularly in cases where low radiation doses limit efficacy of radionuclide therapy alone.[9]

THE CHALLENGE OF PREDICTING RESPONSE TO IMMUNE CHECK-POINT INHIBITORS

The immune environment is extremely complex with multiple cell types involved, complex signaling pathways, and multiple effector mechanisms.[10] The TME is also very important with factors including tissue hypoxia and low pH also influencing the ability of the adaptive immune response to control or eradicate cancer.[11] There has been a great deal of work invested in the search for robust predictive biomarkers of response to ICIs.[12] These have included analysis of blood and tissue factors. Most of these have demonstrated limited capacity for predicting responses in individual patients, especially because these biomarkers can have a heterogeneous spatial and temporal distribution. Despite these limitations, cancers with a high mutational burden, such as melanoma and NSCLC do tend to have a higher response rate.[13] Circulating tumor DNA may provide evidence of high microsatellite instability cancers relating to mismatch repair defects, which has also been shown to increase the likelihood of response to ICIs.[14] There has been significant interest in evaluation of the number and pattern of tumor infiltrating lymphocytes (TILs), which have prognostic significance in some cancers.[15] Immunohistochemistry of tissue specimens for either PD-1 or PD-L1, which have particularly been used in some immunotherapy trials in NSCLC to enrich the population for response, has also shown some promise.[16] However, these techniques currently lack methodologic harmonization and remain primarily experimental.

The need for robust predictive biomarkers is great because the combination of high cost and significant toxicity of ICIs with a low response rate means that neither patients nor society benefits from this treatment in the majority of cases. Consequently, there is increasing interest in imaging biomarkers, particularly those involving specific molecular imaging agents that can noninvasively assess global expression of immune targets serially.[17] These are not yet approved for clinical use and only available in a few sites internationally with specialist radiochemistry capability. With respect to the more routinely accessible technology of FDG PET/CT, a promising predictor of response seems to be tumor burden using a parameter termed whole-body metabolic tumor volume (wbMTV). Analysis tools

providing user-friendly segmentation of disease burden based on FDG uptake are becoming more widely available from both scanner manufacturers and third-party vendors (**Fig. 1**). In a study involving 142 patients treated with ipilumumab, patients with a wMTV above the median for the group had a significantly worse prognosis than those with lower values.[18] Although it might seem self-evident that it would be more difficult to eradicate a large amount of disease, biological factors might also be implicated. These could include the presence of hypoxia in larger disease deposits acting to suppress immune killing or an increased likelihood of resistant clones in a disease with intrinsic genomic instability. The apparent therapeutic benefits of treating a low wbMTV provides a cogent rationale for surveillance of high-risk melanoma using FDG PET/CT. Our group has established such a program based on a Bayesian risk-adapted model wherein patients with smaller volume nodal metastases were imaged at longer intervals and for a longer time than patients with bulkier nodal involvement.[19] In the evaluation of this program, 170 patients underwent FDG PET/CT surveillance and relapses were identified in 38% of patients, of which the majority (69%) were asymptomatic. Patients who had a negative scan at the end of an 18-month surveillance interval had a negative predictive value of 80% to 84% for the various stage III subclasses for lack of recurrence at any time in the median of 47 months of follow-up. A similar approach involving the combination of clinical

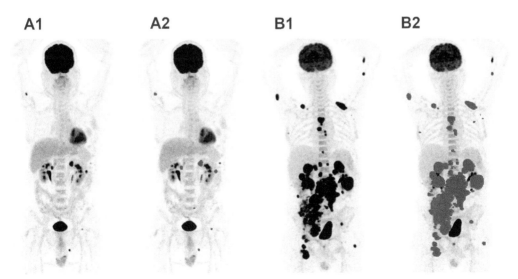

Fig. 1. The wMTV of 2 patients with widely different disease burden. (*A1*) FDG PET maximum intensity projection (MIP) image of a patient with low-volume metastatic melanoma. (*A2*) FDG PET MIP image with tumor segmentation in red with wbMTV of 6 mL. (*B1*) FDG PET MIP of patient with high-volume metastatic melanoma. (*B2*) FDG PET MIP image with tumor segmentation in red and a wbMTV of 1086 mL.

evaluation and blood testing of S100B 3-monthly and 6-monthly FDG PET/CT scans in a small pilot study also demonstrated the ability to detect asymptomatic recurrences.[20] Although the use of adjuvant ICI therapy in patients with fully resected stage III melanoma has improved relapse-free survival,[21] this finding is associated with significant cost and toxicity while only a minority of patients will relapse in the first 12 months after resection without active treatment. We believe that it would be of societal benefit to perform a comparison of active PET surveillance with initiation of ICI at the first evidence of disease relapse versus adjuvant ICI in patients with resected stage III disease evaluating the end points of overall survival, quality of life, and cost utility.

In addition to characteristics of the tumor and its microenvironment, there is increasing interest in the role of microbiome diversity and composition in modulating the immune response. In particular, low levels of gut bacteria and a lack of diversity seem to be associated with lower response rates to cancer immunotherapy.[22] A recent study demonstrated an association between low bacterial load and higher physiologic colonic FDG uptake in healthy human participants,[23] which the authors postulated to reflect a shift in colonic metabolism from short chain fatty acids, produced by colonic bacteria, to glycolysis. They then went on to demonstrate that lower FDG uptake in the colon in a subgroup of patients achieving a complete metabolic response to ipilumumab compared with patients with progressive disease.[24] Whether this factor becomes a reliable predictor of response, particularly in the setting of other ICIs, requires validation in further studies.

THE CHALLENGE OF MONITORING RESPONSE TO IMMUNE CHECK-POINT INHIBITORS

Unlike chemotherapy or radiotherapy, which lead to a reasonably predictable depopulation of cancer cells in responding patients, allowing morphologic measures of response such as the RECIST schema to be used to predict survival[25] or targeted therapies that lead to rapid reduction of glycolytic activity detectable by PET,[26] immunotherapy has increasingly been recognized to have a variety of novel response patterns.[27] These include a temporary increase in apparent tumor burden followed by response, which is termed pseudoprogression and an acceleration of disease, which has been called hyperprogression. Pseudoprogression was first described in melanoma treated with the anti–CTLA-4 agent, ipilumumab, but seems to be a relatively uncommon event,[1] particularly with anti–PD-L1 monotherapy.[28] Hyperprogression is

also uncommon and seems to be primarily related to use of anti–PD-1/PD-L1 agents.[29] The therapeutic consequences of these different modes of response are diametrically opposite. For the first, early cessation of treatment may compromise eventual benefit, whereas for the second, the continuation of treatment may deny patients access to alternative treatments and expose patients to unnecessary cost and toxicity. Enlarging lesions or development of new lesions characterize both and therefore standard RECIST measures fail to differentiate them. This has led to modified various response criteria being proposed for CT scans and MR imaging evaluation of therapeutic response to immunotherapy agents.[30] Although subtly different, each incorporates a need for a follow-up scan to assess whether new lesions continue to progress or regress denying an opportunity for early treatment cessation in cases of hyperprogression.

MECHANISTIC CONSIDERATIONS OF IMMUNE RESPONSE

The immune system plays a critical role in maintaining health by recognizing and responding rapidly to pathogens. It also plays an important role in identifying and killing cancer cells in which mutational changes are expressed as aberrant proteins, termed TAAs. In simplistic terms, the adaptive immune response to cancer involves the interaction between an antigen-presenting cell and T lymphocytes involving the major histocompatibility complex on dendritic cells, TAAs, and the T-cell receptor located on cytotoxic T lymphocytes. This interaction initiates an immune response with both activating and inhibitory limbs, which either promote tumor control or facilitate cancer progression.[31] At the same time as the T-cell receptor is engaged to stimulate an immune response, there is upregulation CTLA-4 and PD-1 in the T lymphocyte, acting as immune checkpoints curtailing this process. The former acts primarily at sites of T-cell priming, which include secondary lymphoid organs such as lymph nodes and the spleen.[10] CTLA-4 also has a role in modulating the behavior of regulator T cells.[32] Expansion and recruitment of cytotoxic T lymphocytes is enhanced by blockade of this immune checkpoint by anti–CTLA-4 antibodies. PD-1 conversely acts primarily within the TME where it engages with PD-L1 on tumor cells to block cell killing. However, PD-L1 is also expressed on various immune suppressive cells including tumor-associated macrophages (TAMs), regulator T cells and myeloid derived suppressor cells (MDSCs). It is suspected that disinhibition of these cells, particularly immune suppressing TAMs, may play a role in the phenomenon of hyperprogression seen with use of anti-PD-1/PD-L1 ICIs.[33]

Beyond the roles of CTLA-4 and PD-1/PD-L1, the immune environment is extremely complex, involving a wide range of cells, receptors, and cytokines.[34] These provide a multitude of potential therapeutic targets, many of which are just beginning to be explored.[35] It is also now recognized that there are several different immune environments that can exist in cancer deposits and that are characterized by specific genomic signatures.[36] The failure of the adaptive immune system to eradicate cancer cells, which can be thought of as immune resistance, has several mechanisms. These can include poor TAA presentation, barriers to T-cell infiltration, lack of T-cell response and suppression of the cell killing capability of T cells.[37] These mechanistic factors impact both the likelihood and pattern of response to ICIs.

IMPLICATIONS OF THE TME AND MECHANISM OF ACTION OF IMMUNE CHECK-POINT INHIBITORS FOR PET IMAGING

Although it is convenient to think of FDG uptake in a primary tumor or metastatic site as representing an aggregation of proliferating cancer cells, it is clear that it represents a much more complex process. The metabolic reprogramming of cancer cells through oncogenic signaling, the effects of hypoxia, and the contribution of stromal cells, particularly those of an inflammatory phenotype, all contribute to the apparent intensity of FDG uptake in lesions. This finding is particularly relevant in the context of the immune microenvironment. Recent data indicate the importance of glycolysis in modulating the behavior of immune infiltrating cells in the TME.[38] Indeed, TAMs have recently been shown to increase hypoxia in the TME and also enhance immune and tumor cell glycolysis, contributing to FDG uptake.[39] Further, PD-L1 expression was recently shown to be significantly correlated with glucose metabolism and hypoxia in NSCLC.[40] In this evaluation of adenocarcinoma, the both PD-L1 expression and maximum standardized uptake value (SUV_{max}) were identified as independent prognostic predictors by multivariate analysis. Despite also demonstrating a positive correlation between SUV_{max} and PD-L1 expression, patients with NSCLC with a high SUV_{max} had a worse rather than better response to nivolumab in a recent preliminary report.[41] An association between SUV_{max} and PD-1/PD-L1 expression has also recently been demonstrated in bladder cancer,[42] a cancer that is also

responsive to immunotherapy. It is, therefore, unclear whether SUV_{max} will be a reliable predictive biomarker of response to anti–PD-L1 ICIs. This is a limitation also of other biomarkers, including serum lactate dehydrogenase levels, which have prognostic value but are not predictive of response to ICIs.[43]

In the setting of therapeutic response assessment, recruitment and activation of T lymphocytes into the TME after treatment with ipilumumab has been shown to contribute to the phenomenon of pseudoprogression and stimulated the initial recommendation for modification of immune response criteria.[44] Infiltrating lymphocytes contribute to FDG uptake and tumor volume and can thereby also confound interpretation of FDG PET/CT scans. However, since the initial expansion and activation of these cells occurs in draining lymph nodes, demonstration of new nodes with increased FDG uptake but benign features on CT scans in the next echelon of nodes draining prior sites of involvement, particularly if there is some regression in prior sites of disease, can be clues to this process.[45] This is often accompanied by an increase in uptake in the spleen (**Fig. 2**). Evaluation of the prognostic significance of these findings in a small cohort of patients receiving ipilumumab for melanoma demonstrated that, although all patients demonstrating a nodal flare, particularly in mediastinal nodes in the context of lung metastases, had apparent clinical benefit from treatment, it was not necessary for therapeutic benefit to be observed.[46] In an early study of the usefulness of FDG PET/CT in monitoring immunotherapy, with the majority (16/20) receiving ipilumumab, an increase of greater than 15.5% in peak SUV corrected for lean body mass (SULpeak) as per PERCIST in patients with otherwise stable disease on RECIST evaluation, was associated with clinical benefit.[47] In a larger and more recent study involving 60 patients with metastatic melanoma treated with ipilumumab, evaluation of response at the end of treatment was performed using SULpeak in 5 lesions was used according to PERCIST5 and well as by imPERCIST5, the latter including evaluation of new lesions without recording these immediately as progressive disease.[48] This demonstrated that relatively few patients (2/60) seemed to have pseudoprogression as indicated by new lesions that resolved with ongoing treatment. Because scans were performed at the end of treatment, the rate of pseudoprogression might have been higher than that reported. Nevertheless, responders on FDG PET/CT scans, as defined by either a complete metabolic response (CMR) or partial metabolic response (PMR) had markedly improved survival

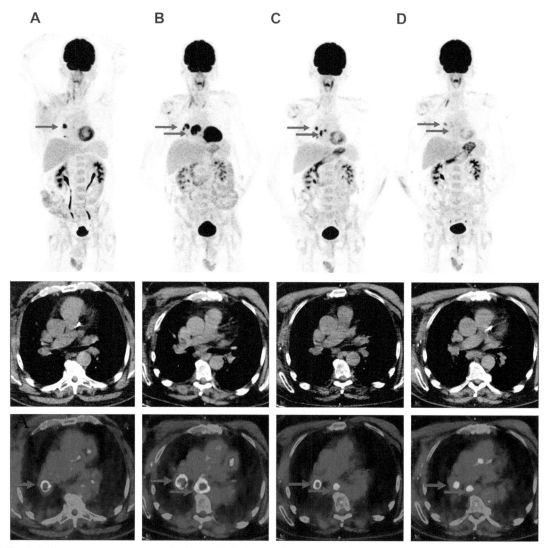

Fig. 2. Early apparent progression in the nodal drainage of metastases after immunotherapy. (*A*) FDG PET MIP, CT scan, and PET/CT scan of a patient with metastatic melanoma involving right lung and right pulmonary hilum (*arrows*). (*B*) FDG PET MIP, CT scan, and PET/CT scan at 2 months after commencement of combination ipilimumab and nivolumab show increase in the size and FDG avidity of the draining lymph nodes in the pulmonary hilar and subcarinal regions (*arrows*). (*C, D*), FDG PET MIP, CT scan, and PET/CT scan at 4 and 7 months show subsequent regression of the FDG-avid lymphadenopathy (*arrows*) with ongoing immunotherapy.

irrespective of the method of response assessment used. Similarly, a retrospective analysis involving 103 patients with FDG PET/CT scans at approximately 1 year after commencing treatment with anti–PD-1 ICI (monotherapy in 67% and combined with anti–CTLA-4 in 31%) demonstrated significantly improved and durable survival in patients achieving a CMR versus non-CMR using the European Organization for Research and Treatment of Cancer (EORTC) response criteria.[49] In CMR patients, the majority of whom had discontinued treatment, 96% had ongoing response.

Again, it is unclear whether earlier imaging may have provided equally robust stratification or allowed a change in therapy. Performing scans after treatment potentially allows a switch or escalation of treatments to be instituted in nonresponders but does not facilitate an early change in management strategy.

Studies evaluating response earlier in treatment are, as yet, very limited. The predictive value of FDG PET/CT scans after completion of 4 doses of ipilimumab in patients with metastatic melanoma, with a mean time between the baseline and the posttherapy scan of 3 months, demonstrated the adverse prognostic significance of new lesions. Patients with more than 4 lesions of any size most accurately differentiated patients without clinical benefit, as classified by disease progression, from those with benefit, which in this study included stable disease as well as partial and complete responses as assessed by a composite clinical evaluation.[50] The larger the size of new lesions, the lower the number of new lesions that was required to identify patients at increased risk of death. From these data, the authors suggested a new set of response criteria, incorporating assessment of the number and size of new lesions, which they called PERCIMT. In the same patient cohort, they subsequently analyzed the predictive value of this schema with the EORTC PET response criteria and found that although the EORTC PET response criteria predicted lack of clinical benefit with high specificity, their PERCIMT criteria better predicted clinical benefit by excluding patients with small and transient new lesions.[51] These data were supported by an earlier study in a smaller subgroup of the same trial in which EORTC PET response after 2 cycles of ipilumumab also predicted clinical benefit.[52] Most recently, the same group has shown the ability of the PERCIMT criteria to predict outcome in 16 patients after 2 cycles of ipilumumab delivered after initial clinical improvement on vemurafenib monotherapy.[53] Whether these new lesions represented a new abnormality in draining nodal basins is unclear.

Data on the use of FDG PET/CT scans for monitoring anti–PD-1/PD-L1 therapy in solid tumors are also limited. In a study of patients with metastatic NSCLC receiving atezolizumab, an anti–PD-L1 ICI, evaluable baseline and at week 6 FDG-PET scans were available in 103 patients.[28] Using the EORTC criteria, patients with an increase in wMTV early during treatment had inferior survival outcome, whereas only 2 patients seemed to have pseudoprogression at this time point. These data suggest that progression on FDG PET/CT scans should generally be considered as true progression unless there are strong clinical indications to the contrary. However, there is a significant caveat to this, which is when the pattern of involvement suggests that development of sarcoidosis, typically with symmetric hilar, mediastinal and often portocaval nodal uptake and sometimes either diffuse or multifocal splenic abnormality (**Fig. 3**). The association of sarcoid-like nodal activation with

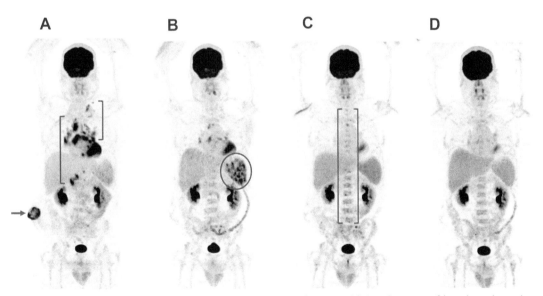

Fig. 3. Dynamic nature of sarcoidosis in response to immunotherapy with involvement of lymph nodes, spleen, and bone marrow. (*A*) FDG PET MIP image of a patient with metastatic melanoma with a flank lesion (*arrow*) after commencement of pembrolizumab shows FDG-avid lymphadenopathy in the mediastinum, bilateral pulmonary hilar, left supraclavicular, and portocaval regions (*brackets*) with mild diffuse uptake in the spleen. (*B*) FDG PET MIP image at 12 months of follow-up shows response in the flank with resolving FDG-avid lymphadenopathy but with increase in multifocal-on-diffuse splenic sarcoid activity (*circle*). (*C*) FDG PET MIP image at 18 months demonstrates resolving splenic activity with increased multifocal-on-diffuse bone marrow activity (*brackets*). (*D*) FDG PET MIP image 1 month after cessation of pembrolizumab depicts resolving bone marrow activity with ongoing CMR.

immune-modulating agents like was recognized for many years ago on gallium-67 citrate imaging.[54] The characteristic lambda pattern of uptake in hilar and mediastinal nodes is a clue to this process. There are now numerous case reports of this process occurring in combination with the use of ICIs.[55] In a further attempt to deal with the possibility of pseudoprogression, another group has proposed an adaptation of the PERCIST criteria that requires confirmation of progressive disease by repeating the FDG PET/CT scan in 4 to 8 weeks. They have called this iPERCIST.[56] They established the preliminary usefulness of these criteria in a cohort of NSCLC patients being treated with nivolumab. In another study involving 49 patients with metastatic melanoma, 16 of whom received ipilumumab and remainder anti–PD-1 ICIs, response was evaluated by comparing FDG PET/CT imaging performed before initiating immunotherapy and after 4 cycles of ICI ipilumumab and pembrolizumab or 6 of nivolumab.[57] In this series, only 1 patient, who had received ipilumumab experienced pseudoprogression and none had hyperprogression. According to PERCIST 1.0, the median overall survival was significantly higher for responders than nonresponders. In our experience, the pattern of metabolic response to anti–PD-1/PD-L1 ICIs in solid tumors is similar to other cytotoxic therapies with a progressive decrease in disease burden, although the rate of response can be quite slow (**Fig. 4**).

In summary, although the current evidence base is scant, given the rarity of pseudoprogression in the setting of ICI treatment, development of new lesions or enlargement of existing lesions should probably be interpreted as progression unless the patient's clinical condition has manifestly improved on treatment. This is particularly the case for anti–PD-1/PD-L1 agents. The rate of pseudoprogression in patients receiving combined anti–CTLA-4/PD-1 (eg, ipilumumab, nivolumab) remains unclear but is also likely to be relatively low.

THE VALUE ADD OF 18F-FLUORODEOXYGLUCOSE POSITRON EMISSION TOMOGRAPHY/COMPUTED TOMOGRAPHY IN RESPONSE ASSESSMENT

Despite the promise of ICI therapy, there is a significant burden of toxicity, which are termed immune-related adverse events (irAE).[58] Because these are generally related to autoimmune phenomena and involve activation of the immune system, these are often readily recognized on FDG PET/CT.[59] Most of these irAE occur relatively early during therapy and can be manifest as inflammatory changes on FDG PET/CT scanning before the onset of symptoms. Almost any organ can be involved but important sites of involvement include the bowel, particularly manifest as colitis, the lungs, endocrine organs, and skin (**Fig. 5**). Rheumatic irAEs can be detected on FDG PET/CT scans and often require prolonged therapy including use of steroids, which could potentially suppress immunity but paradoxically the response rate in a cohort of patients identified with such irAEs, the response rate was higher than expected.[60] In the case of nivolumab monotherapy, the occurrence of irAEs was positively associated with both response and overall survival.[3] Most

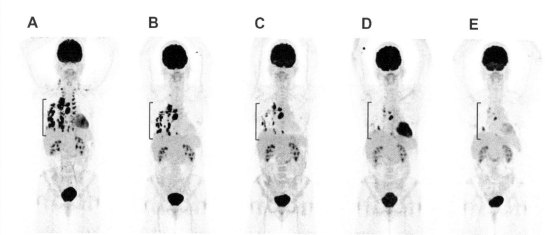

Fig. 4. Slow response to immunotherapy in a patient with metastatic NSCLC. (*A*) FDG PET MIP image shows FDG-avid multifocal metastatic disease in the right thorax (*bracket*). (*B–E*) FDG PET MIP images demonstrate gradual response with ongoing regression of the volume of metastatic disease (*brackets*) at 2 months, 4 months, 7 months, and 9 months, respectively, after commencement of pembrolizumab.

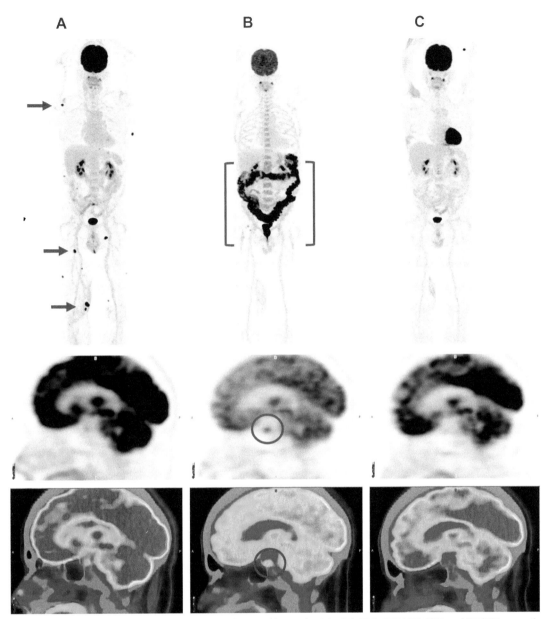

Fig. 5. FDG PET evidence of immune related colitis and hypophysitis. (*A*) FDG PET MIP, PET, and PET/CT scan of a patient with metastatic melanoma show multiple metastases at baseline scan (*arrows*). (*B*) Complete metabolic response with development of intense diffuse uptake in the colon (*brackets*) and pituitary gland (*circle*) after 2 cycles of combination ipilimumab/nivolumab. (*C*) Subsequent resolution of diffuse uptake in the colon and pituitary fossa on follow-up at 3 months.

irAEs are more common with ipilumumab than with anti–PD1-/PD-L1 ICIs, but highest with the combination.[61]

SUMMARY

Despite the encouraging response rates and durability of response in patients deriving clinical benefit from ICIs, many challenges persist in providing prognostic information for patients, selecting patients for treatment with these agents, and knowing when to withdraw or escalate treatment, for example, by adding anti–CTLA-4 treatment to patients with an incomplete response to anti–PD-1 ICI. FDG PET/CT scanning shares some but not all of the limitations of anatomic imaging. Emerging data support its usefulness for monitoring therapeutic response. The optimal timing of response assessment, the most robust interpretation criteria, and whether quantitative or qualitative assessment should be applied remain unclear. The development of new lesions usually but not invariably represents disease progression and careful consideration of clinical factors, anatomic imaging results and the pattern of abnormality are important in identifying poor responders, and changing therapy in a timely manner.

REFERENCES

1. Callahan MK, Wolchok JD, Allison JP. Anti-CTLA-4 antibody therapy: immune monitoring during clinical development of a novel immunotherapy. Semin Oncol 2010;37(5):473–84.
2. Okazaki T, Honjo T. PD-1 and PD-1 ligands: from discovery to clinical application. Int Immunol 2007; 19(7):813–24.
3. Topalian SL, Hodi FS, Brahmer JR, et al. Five-year survival and correlates among patients with advanced melanoma, renal cell carcinoma, or non-small cell lung cancer treated with nivolumab. JAMA Oncol 2019. [Epub ahead of print].
4. Tang J, Shalabi A, Hubbard-Lucey VM. Comprehensive analysis of the clinical immuno-oncology landscape. Ann Oncol 2018;29(1):84–91.
5. Cooper ZA, Frederick DT, Ahmed Z, et al. Combining checkpoint inhibitors and BRAF-targeted agents against metastatic melanoma. Oncoimmunology 2013;2(5):e24420.
6. Gotwals P, Cameron S, Cipolletta D, et al. Prospects for combining targeted and conventional cancer therapy with immunotherapy. Nat Rev Cancer 2017;17(5):286–301.
7. Weichselbaum RR, Liang H, Deng L, et al. Radiotherapy and immunotherapy: a beneficial liaison? Nat Rev Clin Oncol 2017;14(6):365–79.
8. Brooks ED, Chang JY. Time to abandon single-site irradiation for inducing abscopal effects. Nat Rev Clin Oncol 2019;16(2):123–35.
9. Violet JA, Jackson P, Ferdinandus J, et al. Dosimetry of Lu-177 PSMA-617 in metastatic castration-resistant prostate cancer: correlations between pre-therapeutic imaging and "whole body" tumor dosimetry with treatment outcomes. J Nucl Med 2019;60(4):517–23.
10. Wei SC, Duffy CR, Allison JP. Fundamental mechanisms of immune checkpoint blockade therapy. Cancer Discov 2018;8(9):1069–86.
11. Corbet C, Feron O. Tumour acidosis: from the passenger to the driver's seat. Nat Rev Cancer 2017; 17(10):577–93.
12. Havel JJ, Chowell D, Chan TA. The evolving landscape of biomarkers for checkpoint inhibitor immunotherapy. Nat Rev Cancer 2019;19(3): 133–50.
13. Samstein RM, Lee CH, Shoushtari AN, et al. Tumor mutational load predicts survival after immunotherapy across multiple cancer types. Nat Genet 2019;51(2):202–6.
14. Cabel L, Proudhon C, Romano E, et al. Clinical potential of circulating tumour DNA in patients receiving anticancer immunotherapy. Nat Rev Clin Oncol 2018;15(10):639–50.
15. Mlecnik B, Bindea G, Pagès F, et al. Tumor immuno-surveillance in human cancers. Cancer Metastasis Rev 2011;30(1):5–12.
16. Camidge DR, Doebele RC, Kerr KM. Comparing and contrasting predictive biomarkers for immunotherapy and targeted therapy of NSCLC. Nat Rev Clin Oncol 2019;16(6):341–55.
17. Mayer AT, Gambhir SS. The immunoimaging toolbox. J Nucl Med 2018;59(8):1174–82.
18. Ito K, Schöder H, Teng R, et al. Prognostic value of baseline metabolic tumor volume measured on ^{18}F-fluorodeoxyglucose positron emission tomography/computed tomography in melanoma patients treated with ipilimumab therapy. Eur J Nucl Med Mol Imaging 2019;46(4):930–9.
19. Lewin J, Sayers L, Kee D, et al. Surveillance imaging with FDG-PET/CT in the post-operative follow-up of stage 3 melanoma. Ann Oncol 2018;29(7):1569–74.
20. Madu MF, Timmerman P, Wouters MWJM, et al. PET/CT surveillance detects asymptomatic recurrences in stage IIIB and IIIC melanoma patients: a prospective cohort study. Melanoma Res 2017;27(3):251–7.
21. Eggermont AMM, Robert C, Ribas A. The new era of adjuvant therapies for melanoma. Nat Rev Clin Oncol 2018;15(9):535–6.
22. Gopalakrishnan V, Helmink BA, Spencer CN, et al. The influence of the gut microbiome on cancer, immunity, and cancer immunotherapy. Cancer Cell 2018;33(4):570–80.
23. Boursi B, Werner TJ, Gholami S, et al. Functional imaging of the interaction between gut microbiota and the human host: a proof-of-concept clinical study evaluating novel use for 18F-FDG PET-CT. PLoS One 2018;13(2):e0192747.
24. Boursi B, Werner TJ, Gholami S, et al. Physiologic colonic fluorine-18-fluorodeoxyglucose uptake may predict response to immunotherapy in patients with metastatic melanoma. Melanoma Res 2019;29(3):318–21.
25. Therasse P, Eisenhauer EA, Verweij J. RECIST revisited: a review of validation studies on tumour assessment. Eur J Cancer 2006;42(8):1031–9.
26. Van den Abbeele AD, Badawi RD. Use of positron emission tomography in oncology and its potential role to assess response to imatinib mesylate therapy in gastrointestinal stromal tumors (GISTs). Eur J Cancer 2002;38(Suppl 5):S60–5.
27. Borcoman E, Kanjanapan Y, Champiat S, et al. Novel patterns of response under immunotherapy. Ann Oncol 2019;30(3):385–96.

28. Spigel DR, Chaft JE, Gettinger S, et al. FIR: efficacy, safety, and biomarker analysis of a phase II open-label study of atezolizumab in PD-L1-selected patients with NSCLC. J Thorac Oncol 2018;13(11): 1733–42.
29. Champiat S, Ferrara R, Massard C, et al. Hyperprogressive disease: recognizing a novel pattern to improve patient management. Nat Rev Clin Oncol 2018;15(12):748–62.
30. Seymour L, Bogaerts J, Perrone A, et al. iRECIST: guidelines for response criteria for use in trials testing immunotherapeutics. Lancet Oncol 2017; 18(3):e143–52.
31. Barnes TA, Amir E. HYPE or HOPE: the prognostic value of infiltrating immune cells in cancer. Br J Cancer 2017;117(4):451–60.
32. Togashi Y, Shitara K, Nishikawa H. Regulatory T cells in cancer immunosuppression - implications for anticancer therapy. Nat Rev Clin Oncol 2019;16(6): 356–71.
33. Lo Russo G, Moro M, Sommariva M, et al. Antibody-Fc/FcR interaction on macrophages as a mechanism for hyperprogressive disease in non-small cell lung cancer subsequent to PD-1/PD-L1 blockade. Clin Cancer Res 2019;25(3): 989–99.
34. Chen DS, Mellman I. Oncology meets immunology: the cancer-immunity cycle. Immunity 2013;39(1): 1–10.
35. Smyth MJ, Ngiow SF, Ribas A, et al. Combination cancer immunotherapies tailored to the tumour microenvironment. Nat Rev Clin Oncol 2016;13(3): 143–58.
36. Ding L, Bailey MH, Porta-Pardo E, et al. Perspective on oncogenic processes at the end of the beginning of cancer genomics. Cell 2018;173(2): 305–20.e10.
37. Day D, Monjazeb AM, Sharon E, et al. From famine to feast: developing early-phase combination immunotherapy trials wisely. Clin Cancer Res 2017; 23(17):4980–91.
38. Li X, Wenes M, Romero P, et al. Navigating metabolic pathways to enhance antitumour immunity and immunotherapy. Nat Rev Clin Oncol 2019; 16(7):425–41.
39. Jeong H, Kim S, Hong BJ, et al. Tumor-associated macrophages enhance tumor hypoxia and aerobic glycolysis. Cancer Res 2019;79(4):795–806.
40. Kaira K, Shimizu K, Kitahara S, et al. 2-Deoxy-2-[fluorine-18] fluoro-d-glucose uptake on positron emission tomography is associated with programmed death ligand-1 expression in patients with pulmonary adenocarcinoma. Eur J Cancer 2018;101:181–90.
41. Evangelista L, Cuppari L, Menis J, et al. 18F-FDG PET/CT in non-small-cell lung cancer patients: a potential predictive biomarker of response to immunotherapy. Nucl Med Commun 2019;40(8): 802–7.
42. Chen R, Zhou X, Liu J, et al. Relationship between the expression of PD-1/PD-L1 and. Eur J Nucl Med Mol Imaging 2019;46(4):848–54.
43. Jessurun CAC, Vos JAM, Limpens J, et al. Biomarkers for response of melanoma patients to immune checkpoint inhibitors: a systematic review. Front Oncol 2017;7:233.
44. Wolchok JD, Hoos A, O'Day S, et al. Guidelines for the evaluation of immune therapy activity in solid tumors: immune-related response criteria. Clin Cancer Res 2009;15(23):7412–20.
45. Wong AN, McArthur GA, Hofman MS, et al. The advantages and challenges of using FDG PET/CT for response assessment in melanoma in the era of targeted agents and immunotherapy. Eur J Nucl Med Mol Imaging 2017;44(Suppl 1):67–77.
46. Sachpekidis C, Larribère L, Kopp-Schneider A, et al. Can benign lymphoid tissue changes in. Cancer Immunol Immunother 2019;68(2):297–303.
47. Wahl RL, Jacene H, Kasamon Y, et al. From RECIST to PERCIST: evolving considerations for PET response criteria in solid tumors. J Nucl Med 2009; 50(Suppl 1):122S–50S.
48. Ito K, Teng R, Schöder H, et al. F-FDG PET/CT for monitoring of ipilimumab therapy in patients with metastatic melanoma. J Nucl Med 2019;60(3): 335–41.
49. Tan AC, Emmett L, Lo S, et al. FDG-PET response and outcome from anti-PD-1 therapy in metastatic melanoma. Ann Oncol 2018;29(10):2115–20.
50. Anwar H, Sachpekidis C, Winkler J, et al. Absolute number of new lesions on ^{18}F-FDG PET/CT is more predictive of clinical response than SUV changes in metastatic melanoma patients receiving ipilimumab. Eur J Nucl Med Mol Imaging 2018; 45(3):376–83.
51. Sachpekidis C, Anwar H, Winkler J, et al. The role of interim ^{18}F-FDG PET/CT in prediction of response to ipilimumab treatment in metastatic melanoma. Eur J Nucl Med Mol Imaging 2018; 45(8):1289–96.
52. Sachpekidis C, Larribere L, Pan L, et al. Predictive value of early 18F-FDG PET/CT studies for treatment response evaluation to ipilimumab in metastatic melanoma: preliminary results of an ongoing study. Eur J Nucl Med Mol Imaging 2015;42(3):386–96.
53. Sachpekidis C, Kopp-Schneider A, Hakim-Meibodi L, et al. 18F-FDG PET/CT longitudinal studies in patients with advanced metastatic melanoma for response evaluation of combination treatment with vemurafenib and ipilimumab. Melanoma Res 2019;29(2):178–86.
54. Shiomi S, Kuroki T, Yokogawa T, et al. Changes in results of Gallium-67-citrate scanning after interferon

therapy for chronic hepatitis C. J Nucl Med 1997;
38(2):216–9.

55. Reuss JE, Kunk PR, Stowman AM, et al. Sarcoidosis in the setting of combination ipilimumab and nivolumab immunotherapy: a case report & review of the literature. J Immunother Cancer 2016;4:94.

56. Goldfarb L, Duchemann B, Chouahnia K, et al. Monitoring anti-PD-1-based immunotherapy in non-small cell lung cancer with FDG PET: introduction of iPERCIST. EJNMMI Res 2019;9(1):8.

57. Amrane K, Le Goupil D, Quere G, et al. Prediction of response to immune checkpoint inhibitor therapy using 18F-FDG PET/CT in patients with melanoma. Medicine (Baltimore) 2019;98(29):e16417.

58. Postow MA, Sidlow R, Hellmann MD. Immune-related adverse events associated with immune checkpoint blockade. N Engl J Med 2018;378(2):158–68.

59. Aide N, Hicks RJ, Le Tourneau C, et al. FDG PET/CT for assessing tumour response to immunotherapy : report on the EANM symposium on immune modulation and recent review of the literature. Eur J Nucl Med Mol Imaging 2019;46(1):238–50.

60. Mitchell EL, Lau PKH, Khoo C, et al. Rheumatic immune-related adverse events secondary to anti-programmed death-1 antibodies and preliminary analysis on the impact of corticosteroids on anti-tumour response: a case series. Eur J Cancer 2018;105:88–102.

61. Boutros C, Tarhini A, Routier E, et al. Safety profiles of anti-CTLA-4 and anti-PD-1 antibodies alone and in combination. Nat Rev Clin Oncol 2016;13(8):473–86.

Current Evidence on PET Response Assessment to Immunotherapy in Lymphomas

Egesta Lopci, MD, PhD[a], Michel Meignan, MD, PhD[b],*

KEYWORDS

- Hodgkin lymphoma • Immunotherapy • Checkpoint inhibitors • CAR-T • PET/CT • FDG PET
- Response assessment • LYRIC

KEY POINTS

- Response assessment in malignant lymphoma has progressively grown in the last 20 years.
- Rather than asking how useful PET is in a retrospective view, oncologists and imagers should better cooperate in setting clinical trials right away using the most adequate imaging modality and perform in parallel studies on predictive factors, including imaging biomarkers.
- Ongoing trials and future studies represent another chance for both parties to answer questions on clinical needs and optimize collaboration for the sake of patient benefit.

IMMUNOTHERAPY IN LYMPHOMA

Assignment of the Nobel Prize in Physiology or Medicine in 2018 to Allison and Honjo "for their discovery of cancer therapy by inhibition of negative immune regulation"[1] demonstrates the striking relevance of immunomodulating agents in oncology. However, the use of immunotherapy in cancer treatment has a longer history than actually imaginable and can be dated back to the first time William Coley used his microbial product in 1890.[2] Notwithstanding, its real breakthrough arrived with checkpoint inhibitors in 2010 and the first impressive results obtained with ipilimumab, an anti-CTLA-4 (cytotoxic T lymphocyte antigen-4) antibody, in metastatic melanoma.[3] Subsequently, CTLA-4 and the pathway involving the programmed cell death protein 1 (PD-1) and its ligands (PD-L1 and PD-L2) have revolutionized the oncologic scenario in the last decade leading to the approval by the Food and Drug Administration (FDA) and

the European Medicines Agency (EMA) of several monoclonal antibodies. Currently, not only ipilimumab but also nivolumab and pembrolizumab (anti-PD-1), atezolizumab, avelumab, or durvalumab (anti-PD-L1) are used as standard of care for multiple solid tumors.[4] Similar outstanding results have been obtained also for hematologic malignancies,[5–7] especially for relapsed or refractory classical Hodgkin lymphoma (HL). The rationale behind the use of checkpoint inhibitors in HL resides in the same characteristics of Reed-Sternberg cells and lymphoma microenvironment, capable of overexpressing PD-L1 in approximately 70% (range 54%–100%) of the cases.[8,9] The activation of the PD-1/PD-L1 pathway limits T-cell response against cancer and promotes Reed-Sternberg cell growth, helping the tumor evade the immune surveillance.[10–13] The blockade of this inhibitory circuit is expected to interrupt the process and promote immune response against cancer cells. In fact, already during the first preliminary data

Conflicts of Interest: E. Lopci declares research grants from Fondazione AIRC and the Italian Ministry of Health.
[a] Nuclear Medicine Humanitas Clinical and Research Hospitlae IRCCS, Via Manzoni 56 Rozzano, Milan, Italy;
[b] Lysa Imaging, Henri Mondor University Hospitals, APHP, University Paris East, Créteil 94010, France
* Corresponding author.
E-mail address: michel.meignan-ext@aphp.fr

PET Clin 15 (2020) 23–34
https://doi.org/10.1016/j.cpet.2019.08.011

with anti-PD-1 therapy in HL, Ansell and colleagues[5] could report response rates of up to 87% in relapsed or refractory cases treated with nivolumab. Therapeutic efficacy was proved later on also with pembrolizumab used in brentuximab vedotin relapsed HL (KEYNOTE-013), providing an overall response rate of 65%.[6] Thanks to these studies and to other confirmatory ones,[11,14] the anti-PD-1 agents nivolumab and pembrolizumab have been approved as standard treatment in relapsed or refractory HL.

The impact of checkpoint inhibitors for the treatment of other lymphoma types has been less striking compared with HL. A lower and more variable rate of PD-1 and PD-L1 expression in other histologies[9,15] has been noted. For instance, in diffuse large B-cell lymphoma (DLBCL), overexpression of PD-L1 ranges between 14% and 31%.[8,9] Also, response rates result markedly below HL, passing from 10.3% to 36%.[15,16] Consequently, no actual approval exists for checkpoint inhibitors in DLBCL. Nevertheless, immunotherapy represents the mainframe for non-Hodgkin lymphoma (NHL) if the standard regimens applying the monoclonal anti-CD20 antibody rituximab are considered,[17] and more recently the chimeric antigen receptor T (CAR-T) cell therapy[18,19] FDA and EMA approved for adults with relapsed or refractory large B-cell lymphomas (Fig. 1). CAR-T cells are autologous T lymphocytes that have been engineered to express specific receptors targeting antigens associated with cancer.[15] Axicabtagene ciloleucel and Tisagenlecleucel, the 2 approved therapies,[20–23] target CD19 that is expressed on the B-cell surface in case of malignancy and at all differentiation stages.[24] Overall response rates reached from initially treated cohorts quote up to 82%, with a complete response (CR) rate of 54% and a durable disease responsiveness at follow-up.[19] Possible limitations relate to either side effects or costs, which impact the patients' quality of life and the economic sustainability of national health care systems, respectively.[25]

RESPONSE PATTERNS DURING IMMUNOTHERAPY

Immunotherapy has recently gained the above-mentioned remarkable place in cancer treatment not simply as a consequence of the high response rates achieved but also thanks to the durable responses visible after treatment stop or even in case therapy continuation beyond disease progression.[26] This later aspect, reported similarly for solid tumors[27] as well as for hematologic malignancies,[28] introduces additional confusion in response assessment. In fact, one of the peculiarities and potential pitfalls of immunomodulating agents used in cancer concerns response patterns. Besides conventional responses associated with complete or partial regression (Fig. 2), stable and progressive disease, immunotherapy with checkpoint inhibitors has promoted pseudoprogression as part of the therapeutic effect. This new pattern of response to treatment, typically observed in solid tumors under immunotherapy and particularly in melanoma, affects 5% to 12% of the cases.[29] The phenomenon is defined as a transient increase in tumor size secondary to an augmented immune infiltrate. Rather than a real progression, pseudoprogression represents a flare phenomenon induced by the massive recruitment of immune cells into the tumor microenvironment. Being a transitory event, pseudoprogression is

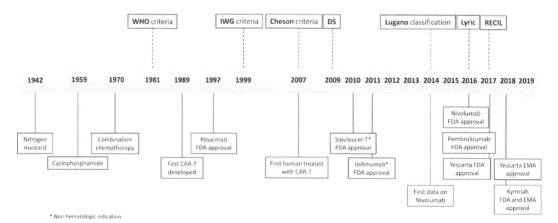

Fig. 1. Timeline of response criteria developed in malignant lymphoma parallel to the evolution of treatment options, focusing primarily on immunotherapy. IWG, international working group; LYRIC, immunomodulatory therapy criteria; WHO, World Health Organization.

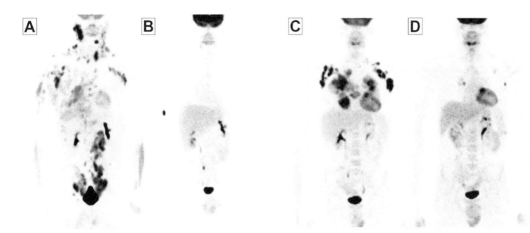

Fig. 2. Pictorial example of 2 patients with HL undergoing immunotherapy with Nivolumab investigated at baseline (A, C) and after 17 weeks of treatment (B, D). These 2 cases display different patterns of response: the first patient on the left (A, B) shows a CMR, despite the extensive tumor burden at baseline; the second patient (C, D) results in a partial responder having some residual metabolically active disease (DS 4) in the left axilla and right pulmonary hilum.

confirmed as such only during subsequent scanning (or in the case of biopsy), demonstrating indeed tumor regression and treatment benefit.[30,31]

Another specific pattern of response first described for immunotherapy is hyperprogression. Hyperprogression affects 4% to 29% of patients and involves in particular the elderly population (age >65 years).[32–34] The key element to define the phenomenon, as initially described by Champiat and colleagues,[32] relies on the tumor growth rate, which in the case of hyperprogression increases at minimum 2-fold between baseline and after therapy initiation. Later on, the timing for assessing hyperprogression could be restricted to 2 months after treatments start.[35] Contrary to pseudoprogression, hyperprogression does not represent a problem for image interpretation, given the usual dramatic tumor growth and clinical worsening, leading in general to a very poor prognosis.[36]

Last, anecdotal reports describe a possible abscopal effect in the course of immunotherapy.[37,38] Being by definition immune mediated, the abscopal effect can determine tumor shrinkage at distant sites of disease following locoregional treatments, typically radiation therapy.

PROPOSED RESPONSE CRITERIA IN LYMPHOMA

Several criteria have been proposed to face the problems of the so-called pseudoprogression (see **Fig. 1**). The Lymphoma response to immunomodulatory therapy criteria (LYRIC) published in 2016[31] have tried to integrate to the Lugano classification dedicated to lymphoma the Immune response criteria previously proposed for solid tumors.[30] They were mainly dedicated to the evaluation of the response to checkpoint inhibitors in HL. Because of the small number of observations, it was considered difficult to identify the different relevant pathophysiologic imaging patterns observed under therapy, which could be of help to eliminate the diagnosis of progression. Therefore, LYRIC classified all of these patterns under the category of indeterminate response (IR), with 3 subcategories: IR1, increase in overall tumor burden (as assessed by sum of product diameters [SPD]) of ≥50% of up to 6 measurable lesions in the first 12 weeks of therapy, without clinical deterioration; IR2, appearance of new lesions, or growth of 1 or more existing lesions ≥50% at any time during treatment occurring in the context of lack of overall progression (<50% increase of overall tumor burden, as measured by SPD of up to 6 lesions); IR3, increase in fludeoxyglucose (FDG) uptake of 1 or more lesions without a concomitant increase in lesion size or number. Importantly, it was also proposed to consider that an increase of FDG avidity of 1 or more lesions suggestive of lymphoma without a concomitant increase in size of those lesions meeting progressive disease (PD) criteria does not constitute PD. These categories were opened to changes using the experience drawn from the clinical observations made under immunomodulatory treatments. LYRIC encouraged biopsy for IR1 and IR2 and advised to evaluate these intermediate features by following up in all cases after 12 weeks by a new scanning in order to judge progression on a basis of an increase of size of greater than 10% for IR1, a new lesion leading to a tumor burden greater than 50% for IR2, or an increase of the lesion size or new lesion for IR3. There is no change between LYRIC and Lugano criteria regarding complete metabolic response (CMR) and partial metabolic response (PMR).

The second group of criteria is the Response evaluation criteria in Lymphoma (RECIL), defined by an international working group in 2017.[39] Contrary to the LYRIC, the objective of RECIL criteria was to homogenize response criteria in trials testing the efficacy of new drugs and including lymphoma and solid tumors. RECIL changed the way to measure the lesions, relying only on unidimensional measurement of the long diameter of 3 selected targets. Contrasting with LYRIC and Lugano criteria, RECIL criteria modified the complete and partial response (PR) categories, decreasing the role of PET. The proposal was based on the observation that some immunomodulatory drugs can alter glucose metabolism, suppressing the existing relationship between the drug efficacy and the FDG uptake observed under chemotherapy. Consequently, the concept of CMR defined in Lugano classification is replaced by CR requiring not only Deauville scoring (DS) 1 to 3 but also at least a 30% reduction of the lesions by computed tomography (CT). PR replaces PMR and implies a 30% reduction of the sum of the longest diameter associated with a positive DS 4 to 5. The objective is to minimize the risk of classifying some of these patients falling in the IR2 category of the LYRIC as PD. To evaluate the effect of agents not fulfilling the criteria for a PR, a third category, named minor response, has been identified with at least a 10% reduction of the tumor burden whatever the PET results. The progression implies a greater than 20% increase of tumor burden or the presence of a new lesion (to put in perspective with the >50% of IR1), whatever the DS. For relapse from CR, at least 1 lesion should measure 2 cm in the long axis. By contrast with LYRIC, RECIL classification does not give recommendation for follow-up of the lesions.

EVIDENCE FROM THE LITERATURE

The first preliminary results on anti-PD-1 therapy in HL were published in December 2014.[5] To assess response to treatment, the investigators used therein a combination of morphologic (CT) and metabolic (FDG PET) data, with the later ones used mainly to confirm CR. Later on, Armand and colleagues[6] reported data on pembrolizumab during the KEYNOTE-013 trial by applying as criteria for response the International Harmonization Project in lymphoma or Cheson 2007 criteria.[40] The same criteria, or their subsequent development,[41] have been variably used also for other immunotherapy trials in HL.[14,28,42–44] Noteworthy, the first dedicated reports on PET response evaluation in lymphoma treated with checkpoint inhibitors were all derived from retrospective analyses. As summarized in **Table 1**, all cases applied Cheson 2014 (or Lugano) criteria for response assessment and compared in parallel (or partially) the results with the proposed LYRIC criteria.[45–47]

The group from Gustave Roussy was the first to describe the kinetics[48] and the patterns of response to immunotherapy.[45] Initially, the investigators analyzed the cohort of 16 patients to assess timing and depth of response to immunotherapy.[48] The investigators report 12.7 months as median time to nadir (range 3–23 months). Within 6 months of treatment, 4 CMR were reported. In 3 cases, CMR was detectable already at 3 months (early evaluation), whereas the fourth converted from PMR to CMR after early evaluation. No other CMR occurred after 6 months of treatment. Of note, 78% of responsive patients at 3 months (3 CMR and 4 PMR) remained in tumor control at 1 year.[48] The same cohort was subsequently analyzed with regards to imaging.[45] In particular, by adopting the DS on a lesion basis (n = 290), response assessment at 3 and 6 months showed a positive predictive value of 88% and 97%, and a negative predictive value of 92% and 97%, respectively. In the study, moreover, all semiquantitative and quantitative variations of PET parameters at 3 months resulted in predictive of the best overall response.

The 5-point scale criteria were considered also in the article from Castello and colleagues.[47] Therein, 43 HL patients treated with anti-PD-1 therapy were enrolled and assessed at 8 weeks (early) and 17 weeks (interim) after treatment start. At early evaluation, performed in 22 patients, visual analysis with DS significantly differentiated responders from nonresponders ($P = .003$).[41] Also, at 17-week evaluation (n = 40), DS was confirmed as significantly different among groups ($P = .008$). By classifying patients at interim evaluation into responders (CR + PR) and nonresponders (stable disease [SD] + PD), the investigators observed a significantly lower risk of progression or death for the first group (hazard ratio 0.13; $P = .01$).

These findings seem to suggest for metabolic response in general, and DS in particular, a predictive role also for immunotherapy with checkpoint inhibitors.[49]

Table 1
Summary of available articles on fludeoxyglucose PET/computed tomographic response evaluation in lymphoma treated with immunotherapy

Authors, Reference	Patients	Study Type	Histology	Treatment	Response Criteria	Results
Dercle et al,[45] 2018	16	Retrospective[a]	HL	Nivolumab (n = 1); Pembrolizumab (n = 15)	Lugano/ LYRIC	Best responses on PET: 6 CR, 4 PR, 2 SD, 4 PD. LYRIC IR were observed in 7 patients, 5 were confirmed PD Responders had increased spleen metabolism at 3 mo
Dercle et al,[48] 2018	16	Retrospective[a]	HL	Nivolumab (n = 1); Pembrolizumab (n = 15)	Lugano/ LYRIC	78% of patients classified as responders at 3 mo remained in tumor control at 1 y. CMR occurred within 6 mo
Rossi et al,[46] 2018	30	Retrospective	HL	Nivolumab (n = 26); Pembrolizumab (n = 4)	Lugano/ LYRIC	Best response: 5 CR, 17 PR, 2 SD, and 6 PD DS 4 and 5 by Lugano (n = 15) were reclassified by LYRIC as PR (n = 4), IR1 (n = 2), IR2 (n = 8), and IR3 (n = 1)
Castello et al,[47] 2019	43	Retrospective	HL	Nivolumab (n = 42); Pembrolizumab (n = 1)	Lugano/ LYRIC	Best clinical responses: 26 CR, 5 PR, 8 SD, and 4 PD. LYRIC reclassified 3 IR1, whereas the last PD case was confirmed. At interim, DS well-differentiated responders from nonresponders
Shah et al,[50] 2018	7	Prospective	3 DLBCL, 4 FL	CAR-T (CTL019)	DS/ Lugano	Responses at 1 mo: 3 CR, 2 PR, and 2 PD
Wang et al,[51] 2019	19	Retrospective	14 DLBCL, 3 FL	CD19-targeting CAR-T	PERCIST	Best overall responses: 7 CR, 8 PR. Possible pseudoprogression in 3. CRS (grade 0–2) had significantly lower MTV and TLG than those with severe CRS (grade 3–4)

Abbreviations: LYRIC, immunomodulatory therapy criteria; PD, 0 progressive disease.
[a] Same study population analyzed with two different ways.

When comparing Lugano criteria with LYRIC, Dercle and colleagues[45] outlined 7 patients with IR, of which 5 cases (71%) were confirmed as PD, whereas only 2 turned out to be pseudo-progression.[45] In the study from Lysa centers,[46] instead, only tangentially comparing the 2 response criteria, the DS 4 and 5 assessed with Lugano criteria (15/30 patients) were reclassified by LYRIC as PR (27%) or IR: IR1 (13%), IR2 (53%), and IR3 (7%). More consistent data were obtained by contrast from Castello and colleagues.[47] In particular, no significant differences were detected between the 2 response criteria, although 3 out of 4 PD patients were reclassified as IR1 according to LYRIC. Given the retrospective nature of all these studies, the clinical utility for new LYRIC criteria appears plausible but not thoroughly proved yet.

More embryonal data exist for CAR-T cell therapy and metabolic response (see **Table 1**). Two separate articles analyze the imaging predictive role by focusing on either early response assessment[50] or side effects.[51] In the first case, Shah and colleagues[50] prospectively analyzed early PET/CT in patients with DLBCL and follicular lymphoma (FL) undergoing CTL019 CAR-T cells. Imaging was obtained 1 month after therapy and response assessment based on DS (Lugano criteria). Their preliminary data published as a correspondence letter on the first 7 patients document 3 CR, 2 PR, and 2 PD at early stage. All complete responders (DS 1 + 2) remained in remission for more than 2 years after the end of therapy, whereas the others progressed. The second article on CAR-T, instead, retrospectively analyzed 17 NHL (14 DLBCL and 3 FL) aiming to define useful semiquantitative and quantitative parameters for prediction of adverse events.[51] Response to therapy was once again assessed at 1 month, but differently from all previously reported articles, it was based on PERCIST (PET Response Criteria in Solid Tumors).[52] Along with CR and PR, the investigators observed 3 cases of pseudoprogression related to local inflammation following the CAR-T effect. Interestingly, high metabolic burden at baseline, that is, metabolic tumor volume (MTV) and total lesion glycolysis (TLG) could predict severe CRS (grade 3 + 4). In particular, median MTV was 49.3 cm^3 versus 1137.7 cm^3 ($P = .012$), and median TLG was 379.1 versus 9384 ($P = .012$), respectively, for mild/moderate CRS versus severe CRS. Larger cohorts are welcome (**Table 2**) to confirm the promising results reported from these articles, it is hoped, for better harmonizing response criteria also for CAR-T therapy.

IMMUNE-RELATED ADVERSE EVENTS

Adverse events are crucial aspects to be taken into account for all oncologic regimens. In accordance with the type of drug administered, the dose, and the duration of therapy, the related adverse events can vary significantly and impact the performance and the quality of patient's life at different grades. With the latest revolution brought forward by immunotherapy in oncology, immune-related adverse events (IAEs) have consequently emerged even more prepotently and are considered major limitations to therapeutic prosecution and a handicap for response assessment (**Fig. 3**). Therefore, it is mandatory for both imagers and clinicians to be aware of their manifestations, timing, and potential differential diagnoses. Notwithstanding, when considering numbers, IAEs are less debilitating and better tolerated compared with toxic side effects secondary to conventional therapies.[53] In fact, in a pooled metaanalysis in advanced solid tumors, by comparing 3450 patients from 7 randomized clinical trials (RCTs), Nishijima and colleagues[53] documented a significantly lower risk of any all-grade and high-grade (grade III–IV) adverse event during PD-1/PD-L1 inhibitors compared with chemotherapy. The overall corresponding incidences were 67.6% versus 82.9% (any all grade), and 11.4% versus 35.7% (high grade), respectively. By contrast, the investigators report a higher risk for rash, pruritus, colitis, aminotransferase elevations, thyroid disease, and pneumonitis during checkpoint inhibitors, typically representing side effects related to the immune modulation. In the case of hematologic malignancies, IAEs seem to occur in most patients treated with nivolumab or pembrolizumab,[5,54] although high-grade IAEs interest 10% to 11% of the patients, with grade 3 to 4 events being represented by pancreatitis, hepatitis, and diarrhea. Thanks to the metabolic assessment with FDG PET/CT, most abovementioned events can be easily depicted and should be promptly reported, because they can be visible before any clinical manifestation.

Although potentially occurring at any time during treatment, IAEs tend to be more frequent after the first 2 to 3 months of therapy. This aspect is a direct consequence of immune system activation. Therefore, IAEs can be considered the undesirable proof that immunotherapy is actually doing what is expected.[55] In this regard, a predictive and prognostic role for IAEs during checkpoint inhibitors and a direct association to therapeutic benefit have been reported.[45,56,57] First, Haratani and colleagues[56] revealed that in patients with non–small cell lung cancer treated

Table 2
Clinical trials[a] evaluating fludeoxyglucose PET/computed tomography in lymphoma treated with immunotherapy

Identifier	Phase	Official Title	Histology	Treatment	Estimated Participants	Imaging Timing	Sponsor	Status
NCT02476734	Early phase 1	A Pilot Study Using FDG-PET/CT Imaging as an Early Predictor of Disease Response in Lymphoma Subjects Receiving Redirected Autologous CART-19 T-cell Immunotherapy	DLBCL, FL	CART-19 autologous T cells	8	6 wk and 1 mo after infusion	University of Pennsylvania	Completed
NCT03086954	Phase 1	Open, Single Arm, Multicenter Phase 2 Clinical Study to Evaluating the Efficacy and Safety of the Chimeric Antigen Receptor T Cell Immunotherapy (CAR-T) for CD19 Positive Lymphoma	CD19-positive NHL	CAR-T	24	90 d after CAR-T	Sinobioway Cell Therapy Co, Ltd	Not yet recruiting
NCT03703050	Phase 2	Phase II Trial of Nivolumab for Pediatric and Adult Relapsing/Refractory ALK + Anaplastic Large Cell Lymphoma, for Evaluation of Response in Patients With Progressive Disease (Cohort 1) or as Consolidative Immunotherapy in Patients in Complete Remission After Relapse (Cohort 2)	ALK + anaplastic large cell lymphoma	Nivolumab	38	24 wk of induction	Gustave Roussy, Cancer Campus, Grand Paris	Recruiting

(continued on next page)

Table 2
(continued)

Identifier	Phase	Official Title	Histology	Treatment	Estimated Participants	Imaging Timing	Sponsor	Status
NCT03038672	Phase 2–RCT	A Randomized Phase 2 Study of CDX-1127 (Varlilumab) in Combination With Nivolumab in Patients With Relapsed or Refractory Aggressive B-Cell Lymphomas	Relapsed or refractory aggressive B-cell lymphomas	Nivolumab with or without varlilumab	106	Up to 2 y	National Cancer Institute	Recruiting
NCT03498612	Phase 2	Phase II Window Study of Pembrolizumab in Untreated B-Cell Non-Hodgkin Lymphoproliferative Diseases	B-cell NHL; FL; indolent HNL; marginal zone lymphoma	Pembrolizumab	33	After 6 cycles	University of Washington	Recruiting

[a] Trials not considering PET imaging for immunotherapy with checkpoint inhibitors or CAR-T cells have been removed from the list.
Data from https://clinicaltrials.gov/; keywords: PET, immunotherapy | lymphoma.

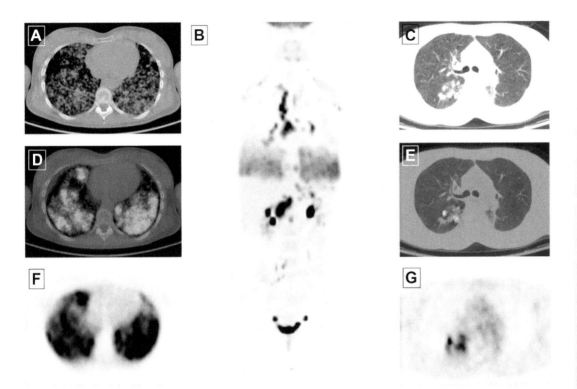

Fig. 3. Different lung involvement in patients with HL undergoing immunotherapy. On the left panels (*A, B, D, F*), a massive parenchymal carcinomatosis is shown, along with multiple nodal involvement in the supradiaphragmatic and infradiaphragmatic regions. On the right side (*C, E, G*), axial views show the appearance of immune-related pneumonitis after 3 months of Nivolumab; the parenchymal consolidation regressed subsequently, and when biopsied, proved to be inflammatory infiltrate.

with Nivolumab (n = 134), the overall response rate was significantly higher in patients with IAEs than in those without (52.3% vs 27.9%, respectively). When using a 6-week landmark analysis, the investigators also showed that IAEs were significantly associated with increased progression-free survival and overall survival. In HL patients treated with anti-PD-1 regimen (n = 16), the reported sign of immune system activation related to response resulted in being the splenic metabolism.[45] In particular, an increase in healthy splenic maximum standardized uptake value (SUV$_{max}$) at 3 months could predict the best overall response. More recently, in another mixed group analysis, comprising melanoma (n = 21), lymphoma (n = 11), and renal cell carcinoma (n = 8), Nobashi and colleagues[57] showed that early occurrence of thyroiditis could anticipate early response to immunotherapy. Differently from Dercle and colleagues,[45] the later article of the group from Stanford[57] reported any decrease of SUV$_{max}$ in the spleen to be associated with clinical benefit. Herein, 82% of the patients developing IAEs had a CR to treatment and, in 7 out of 11 cases, the presence

of IAEs could be revealed only by means of FDG PET scan.[57]

For CAR-T cell therapy in B-cell lymphoma, the situation is somehow different. At first, this therapeutic regimen is associated with other adverse effects, such as cytokine release syndrome (CRS), CAR-T cell-related neurologic toxicities, and B-cell aplasia, not commonly detectable with FDG PET.[51,58–60] Second, concurrent local inflammation is more frequently seen compared with the IAEs mentioned earlier for HL. Last, but not least, adverse events occur quite early after CAR-T therapy administration, that is, hours or days after the first infusion, whereas late side effects are not properly documented.[60] In literature, simple case reports and more recently a retrospective case series[51,60,61] have so far described the appearance of delayed adverse events, also by means of FDG PET/CT.[51,60]

SUMMARY

In a recent expert opinion report,[13] one of the "burning" questions pointed out by the investigator consisted of the effective utility of PET scans in HL undergoing immunotherapy. The answer provided was that PET is less accurate in this context compared with what was expected during chemotherapy[49] and that should not be used outside of clinical trials.[13] The observation is somehow correct, although, considering the small amount of publications available and the lack of coherence in applying response criteria, it should be better to say that there are no sufficient data to make any conclusion. The principle applies to any other imaging modality used to assess response in the case of new treatments types. In fact, CT has not demonstrated to be foolproof in solid tumors treated with immunotherapy,[30,62] and one should not expect it to be better than PET, especially for HL, given the well-known superiority of metabolic imaging over morphology in this malignancy.[40,41] Maybe, rather than asking how useful PET is in a retrospective view, oncologists and imagers should better cooperate in setting clinical trials right away using the most adequate imaging modality and performing in parallel studies on predictive factors, including imaging biomarkers. The ongoing trials (see **Table 2**) and future studies represent another chance for both parties to answer questions on clinical needs and optimize collaboration for the sake of patient benefit.

REFERENCES

1. The Nobel Prize in Physiology or Medicine 2018. NobelPrize.org. Nobel Media AB 2019. 2019. Available at: https://www.nobelprize.org/prizes/medicine/2018/summary/.
2. Nauts H, Fowler G, Bogatko F. A review of the influence of bacterial infection and of bacterial products (Coley's toxins) on malignant tumors in man; a critical analysis of 30 inoperable cases treated by Coley's mixed toxins, in which diagnosis was confirmed by microscopic examination selected for special study. Acta Med Scand Suppl 1953; 276:1–103.
3. Hodi FS, O'Day SJ, McDermott DF, et al. Improved survival with ipilimumab in patients with metastatic melanoma. N Engl J Med 2010; 363:711–23.
4. Rossi S, Toschi L, Castello A, et al. Clinical characteristics of patient selection and imaging predictors of outcome in solid tumors treated with checkpoint-inhibitors. Eur J Nucl Med Mol Imaging 2017;44: 2310–25.
5. Ansell SM, Lesophin AM, Borrello I, et al. PD-1 blockade with nivolumab in relapsed or refractory Hodgkin's lymphoma. N Engl J Med 2015;372: 311–9.
6. Armand P, Shipp M, Ribrag V, et al. Programmed death-1 blockade with pembrolizumab in patients with classical Hodgkin lymphoma after brentuximab vedotin failure. J Clin Oncol 2016;34(31):3733–9.
7. Ansell SM. Targeting immune checkpoints in lymphoma. Curr Opin Hematol 2015;22:337–42.
8. Cheah CY, Fowler NH, Neepalu SS. Targeting the programmed death-1/programmed death-ligand 1 axis in lymphoma. Curr Opin Oncol 2015;27(5): 384–91.
9. Menter T, Bodmer-Haecki A, Dirnhofer S, et al. Evaluation of the diagnostic and prognostic value of PD-L1 expression in Hodgkin and B-cell lymphomas. Hum Pathol 2016;54:17–24.
10. Yamamoto R, Nishikori M, Kitawaki T, et al. PD-1–PD-1 ligand interaction contributes to immunosuppressive microenvironment of Hodgkin lymphoma. Blood 2008;111:3220–4.
11. Younes A, Santoro A, Shipp M, et al. Nivolumab for classical Hodgkin's lymphoma after failure of both autologous stem-cell transplantation and brentuximab vedotin: a multicentre, multicohort, single-arm phase 2 trial. Lancet Oncol 2016;17(9):1283–94.
12. Jalali S, Price-Troska T, Bothun C, et al. Reverse signaling via PD-L1 supports malignant cell growth and survival in classical Hodgkin lymphoma. Blood Cancer J 2019;19:22.
13. Ansell SM. The highs and lows of immune-checkpoint blockade in lymphoma. Cancer Immunol Res 2019;7(5):696–700.
14. Chen R, Zinzani PL, Fanale MA, et al. Phase II study of the efficacy and safety of pembrolizumab for relapsed/refractory classic Hodgkin lymphoma. J Clin Oncol 2017;35(19):2125–32.
15. Zhang J, Medeiros JL, Young KH. Cancer immunotherapy in diffuse large B-cell lymphoma. Front Oncol 2018;8:351.
16. Lesokhin AM, Ansell SM, Armand P, et al. Nivolumab in patients with relapsed or refractory hematologic malignancy: preliminary results of a phase Ib study. J Clin Oncol 2016;34:2698–704.
17. Leget GA, Czuczman MS. Use of rituximab, the new FDA-approved antibody. Curr Opin Oncol 1998; 10(6):548–51.
18. Schuster SJ, Svoboda J, Nasta S, et al. Phase IIa trial of chimeric antigen receptor modified T cells directed against CD19 (CTL019) in patients with relapsed or refractory CD19+ lymphomas. J Clin Oncol 2015;33:8516.
19. Neelapu SS, Locke FL, Bartlett NL, et al. Axicabtagene ciloleucel CAR T-cell therapy in refractory large B-cell lymphoma. N Engl J Med 2017;377(26): 2531–44.
20. U.S. Food & Drug Administration: YESCARTA (axicabtagene ciloleucel). 2017. Available at: https://www.fda.gov/BiologicsBloodVaccines/CellularGeneTherapyProducts/ApprovedProducts/ucm581222.htm.

21. U.S. Food & Drug Administration: KYMRIAH (tisagenlecleucel). 2017. Available at: https://www.fda.gov/biologicsbloodvaccines/cellulargenetherapyproducts/approvedproducts/ucm573706.htm.

22. Axicabtagene ciloleucel, applications for new human medicines under evaluation by the Committee for Medicinal Products for Human Use (EMA/583158/2017). 2017. Available at: http://www.ema.europa.eu/ema/index.jsp?curl=pages/medicines/document_listing/document_listing_000349.jsp&mid=WC0b01ac05805083eb.

23. Tisagenlecleucel, applications for new human medicines under evaluation by the Committee for Medicinal Products for Human Use (EMA/789956/2017). 2017. Available at: http://www.ema.europa.eu/ema/index.jsp?curl=pages/medicines/document_listing/document_listing_000349.jsp&mid=WC0b01ac05805083eb.

24. Tedder TF, Zhou LJ, Engel P. The CD19/CD21 signal transduction complex of B lymphocytes. Immunol Today 1994;15:437–42.

25. Hernandez I, Prasad V, Gellad WF. Total costs of chimeric antigen receptor T-cell immunotherapy. JAMA Oncol 2018;4(7):994–6.

26. Neti N, Esfahani K, Johnson NA. The role of immune checkpoint inhibitors in classical Hodgkin lymphoma. Cancers (Basel) 2018;10(6):204.

27. Borcoman E, Nandikolla A, Long G, et al. Patterns of response and progression to immunotherapy. Am Soc Clin Oncol Educ Book 2018;38:169–78.

28. Armand P, Engert A, Younes A, et al. Nivolumab for relapsed/refractory classic Hodgkin lymphoma after failure of autologous hematopoietic cell transplantation: extended follow-up of the multicohort single-arm phase II CheckMate 205 trial. J Clin Oncol 2018;36(14):1428–39.

29. Chiou VL, Burotto M. Pseudoprogression and immune-related response in solid tumors. J Clin Oncol 2015;33:3541–3.

30. Wolchok JD, Hoos A, O'Day S, et al. Guidelines for the evaluation of immune therapy activity in solid tumors: immune-related response criteria. Clin Cancer Res 2009;15(23):7412–20.

31. Cheson BD, Ansell S, Schwartz L, et al. Refinement of the Lugano classification response criteria for lymphoma in the era of immunomodulatory therapy. Blood 2016;128:2489–96.

32. Champiat S, Dercle L, Ammari S, et al. Hyperprogressive disease (HPD) is a new pattern of progression in cancer patients treated by anti-PD-1/PD-L1. Clin Cancer Res 2017;23:1920–8.

33. Ferrara R, Mezquita L, Texier M, et al. Hyperprogressive disease in patients with advanced non-small cell lung cancer treated with PD-1/PD-L1 inhibitors or with single-agent chemotherapy. JAMA Oncol 2018;4(11):1543–52.

34. Onesti CE, Freres P, Jerusalem G. Atypical patterns of response to immune checkpoint inhibitors: interpreting pseudoprogression and hyperprogression in decision making for patients' treatment. J Thorac Dis 2019;11(1):35–8.

35. Kato S, Goodman A, Walavalkar V, et al. Hyperprogressors after immunotherapy: analysis of genomic alterations associated with accelerated growth rate. Clin Cancer Res 2017;23:4242–50.

36. Saâda-Bouzid E, Defaucheux C, Karabajakian A, et al. Hyperprogression during anti-PD-1/PD-L1 therapy in patients with recurrent and/or metastatic head and neck squamous cell carcinoma. Ann Oncol 2017;28(7):1605–11.

37. Michot JM, Mazeron R, Dercle L, et al. Abscopal effect in a Hodgkin lymphoma patient treated by an anti-programmed death 1 antibody. Eur J Cancer 2016;66:91–4.

38. Ribeiro Gomes J, Schemerling RA, Haddad CK, et al. Analysis of the abscopal effect with anti-PD1 therapy in patients with metastatic solid tumors. J Immunother 2016;39(9):367–72.

39. Younes A, Hilden P, Coiffier B, et al. International Working Group consensus response evaluation criteria in lymphoma. Ann Oncol 2017;28(7):1436–47.

40. Cheson BD, Pfistner B, Juweid ME, et al. International Harmonization Project on Lymphoma. Revised response criteria for malignant lymphoma. J Clin Oncol 2007;25(5):579–86.

41. Cheson BD, Fisher RI, Barrington SF, et al. Recommendations for initial evaluation, staging, and response assessment of Hodgkin and non-Hodgkin lymphoma: the Lugano classification. J Clin Oncol 2014;32(27):3059–68.

42. Moskowitz CH, Zinzani PL, Fanale MA, et al. Pembrolizumab in relapsed/refractory classical Hodgkin lymphoma: primary end point analysis of the phase II keynote-087 study. Blood 2016;128:1107.

43. Maruyama D, Hatake K, Kinoshita T, et al. Multicenter phase II study of nivolumab in Japanese patients with relapsed or refractory classical Hodgkin lymphoma. Cancer Sci 2017;108:1007–12.

44. Chan TSY, Luk TH, Lau JSM, et al. Low-dose pembrolizumab for relapsed/refractory Hodgkin lymphoma: high efficacy with minimal toxicity. Ann Hematol 2017;96:647–51.

45. Dercle L, Seban RD, Lazarovici J, et al. 18F-FDG PET and CT scans detect new imaging patterns of response and progression in patients with Hodgkin lymphoma treated by anti-programmed death 1 immune checkpoint inhibitor. J Nucl Med 2018;59:15–24.

46. Rossi C, Gilhodes J, Maerevoet M, et al. Efficacy of chemotherapy or chemo-anti-PD-1 combination after failed anti-PD-1 therapy for relapsed and

refractory Hodgkin lymphoma: a series from IYsa centers. Am J Hematol 2018;93:1042–9.

47. Castello A, Grizzi F, Qehajaj D, et al. 18F-FDG PET/CT for response assessment in Hodgkin lymphoma undergoing immunotherapy with checkpoint inhibitors. Leuk Lymphoma 2019;6(2):367–75.

48. Dercle L, Ammari S, Seban RD, et al. Kinetics and nadir of responses to immune checkpoint blockade by anti-PD1 in patients with classical Hodgkin lymphoma. Eur J Cancer 2018;91:136–44.

49. Lopci E, Meignan M. Deauville score: the Phoenix rising from ashes. Eur J Nucl Med Mol Imaging 2019;46(5):1043–5.

50. Shah NN, Nagle SJ, Torgian DA, et al. Early positron emission tomography/computed tomography as a predictor of response after CTL019 chimeric antigen receptor-T-cell therapy in B-cell non-Hodgkin lymphomas. Cytotherapy 2018;20:1415–8.

51. Wang J, Hu Y, Yang S, et al. Role of fluorodeoxyglucose positron emission tomography/computed tomography in predicting the adverse effects of chimeric antigen receptor T cell therapy in patients with non-Hodgkin lymphoma. Biol Blood Marrow Transplant 2019;25:1092–8.

52. Wahl RL, Jacene H, Kasamon Y, et al. From RECIST to PERCIST: evolving considerations for PET response criteria in solid tumors. J Nucl Med 2009;50(Suppl 1):122S–50S.

53. Nishijima TF, Shachar SS, Nyrop KA, et al. Safety and tolerability of PD-1/PD-L1 inhibitors compared with chemotherapy in patients with advanced cancer: a meta-analysis. Oncologist 2017;22(4):470–9.

54. Brave M, Liu J, Przepiorka D, et al. Analysis of immune-related adverse reactions in patients with classical Hodgkin lymphoma (cHL) on programmed death-1 (PD-1) inhibitors therapy. Blood 2018;132:1652.

55. Sznol M, Longo D. Release the hounds! Activating the T-cell response to cancer. N Engl J Med 2015;372:374–5.

56. Haratani K, Hayashi H, Chiba Y, et al. Association of immune-related adverse events with nivolumab efficacy in non-small-cell lung cancer. JAMA Oncol 2018;4(3):374–8.

57. Nobashi T, Baratto L, Reddy SA, et al. Predicting response to immunotherapy by evaluating tumors, lymphoid cell-rich organs, and immune-related adverse events using FDG-PET/CT. Clin Nucl Med 2019;44:e272–9.

58. Brudno JN, Kochenderfer JN. Toxicities of chimeric antigen receptor T cells: recognition and management. Blood 2016;127:3321–30.

59. Neelapu SS, Tummala S, Kebriaei P, et al. Chimeric antigen receptor T-cell therapy—assessment and management of toxicities. Nat Rev Clin Oncol 2018;15:47–62.

60. Hu Y, Wang J, Pu C, et al. Delayed terminal ileal perforation in a relapsed/refractory B-cell lymphoma patient with rapid remission following chimeric antigen receptor T-cell therapy. Cancer Res Treat 2018;50(4):1462–6.

61. Wang Y, Zhang WY, Han QW, et al. Effective response and delayed toxicities of refractory advanced diffuse large B-cell lymphoma treated by CD20-directed chimeric antigen receptor-modified T cells. Clin Immunol 2014;155:160–75.

62. Tazdait M, Mezquita L, Lahmar J, et al. Patterns of responses in metastatic NSCLC during PD-1 or PDL-1 inhibitor therapy: comparison of RECIST 1.1, irRECIST and iRECIST criteria. Eur J Cancer 2018;88:38–47.

Programmed Cell Death-1/ Ligand-1 PET Imaging
A Novel Tool to Optimize Immunotherapy?

Sarah R. Verhoeff, MD[a], Michel M. van den Heuvel, MD, PhD[b],
Carla M.L. van Herpen, MD, PhD[a], Berber Piet, MD[b],
Erik H.J.G. Aarntzen, MD, PhD[c], Sandra Heskamp, MD, PhD[c],*

KEYWORDS

- PD-1 • PD-L1 • Cancer • Molecular imaging • immunoPET • Immunotherapy
- Checkpoint inhibitors

KEY POINTS

- Immune checkpoint inhibitors (ICIs) targeting programmed cell death-1/programmed cell death ligand-1 (PD-1/PD-L1) have shown promising results in patients with various advanced stage solid tumors; however, response is limited to a subset of patients.
- Although the number of clinical studies with ICIs is rapidly increasing, there is still an unmet need for a robust biomarker to optimize response.
- PD-1/PD-L1 imaging using radiolabeled antibodies allows in vivo quantification of whole-body PD-1/PD-L1.
- Clinical PD-1/PD-L1 imaging can contribute to a better understanding of the dynamic complexity of PD-1/PD-L1 in the tumor microenvironment.

INTRODUCTION
Programmed Cell Death-1/Programmed Cell Death Ligand-1 Immune Checkpoint Inhibitors

Immune checkpoint inhibitors (ICIs) targeting the programmed cell death (ligand)-1 (PD-[L]1) axis have emerged at the forefront of cancer treatment.[1] Numerous ICIs have received Food and Drug Administration (FDA) and European Medicines Agency (EMA) approval as first-line or second-line treatment in patients with relapsed or metastatic malignancies, including non–small-cell lung cancer (NSCLC),[2–4] melanoma,[5,6] head and neck cancer,[4,7] Merkel cell carcinoma,[8] renal cell carcinoma,[9] and urothelial cell cancer.[10–12]

Currently, indications are rapidly expanding, including in the neo-adjuvant setting.[13]

Two key factors that determine success of ICI are the presence of PD-L1 and infiltration of distinct immune cell populations in the tumor microenvironment.[14–18] Their dynamic and mobile nature highlights the complexity of ICI response. So far, favorable responses have been associated with high tumor PD-L1 expression and high T-cell infiltration. Despite promising clinical results, still only a subset of patients show durable responses to ICI targeting PD-1/PD-L1 and objective response rates are limited to 20% to 40% of patients.[1]

Disclosure statement: All authors declare that there is no conflict of interest.
Funding: Netherlands Organisation for Scientific Research (NWO, project number 91617039), Dutch Cancer Society (KWF, project number 10099), Radboud Institute Health Science (RIHS, project number R0003629).
[a] Department of Medical Oncology, Radboud University Medical Center, Postbus 9101, Nijmegen 6500 HB, the Netherlands; [b] Department of Pulmonary Diseases, Radboud University Medical Center, Postbus 9101, Nijmegen 6500 HB, the Netherlands; [c] Department of Radiology and Nuclear Medicine, Radboud University Medical Center, Postbus 9101, Nijmegen 6500 HB, the Netherlands
* Corresponding author.
E-mail address: Sandra.heskamp@radboudumc.nl

PET Clin 15 (2020) 35–43
https://doi.org/10.1016/j.cpet.2019.08.008

The immune histochemical analysis (IHC) of tumor PD-L1 expression currently is the only registered biomarker for treatment selection.[13–15] It must be noted that patients with tumors stained negative for PD-L1 on a tumor biopsy can benefit from ICI.[2,3] Thus, there is a need for a robust marker for ICI response.[19] In this review, we focus on the prospect of clinical PD-1/PD-L1 imaging studies using radiolabeled antibodies as a tool to predict ICI response and improve our understanding of the tumor microenvironment to optimize the use of ICI.[20]

Programmed Cell Death Ligand-1 Expression as a Marker for Immune Checkpoint Inhibitor Response

The association between high PD-L1 expression in the tumor and ICI response has resulted in the recommendation of the FDA/EMA to restrict the use of pembrolizumab (eg, as first-line treatment for advanced or metastasized NSCLC) to patients with a PD-L1 expressing tumors as assessed by IHC.[2] However, the IHC assessment of PD-L1 on tumor biopsies has several limitations that comprise its clinical use.

First, PD-L1 assessment using IHC on biopsies or single tissue specimen is limited by the heterogeneous tissue expression of PD-L1.[21] This has been illustrated by heterogenic PD-L1 expression between primary tumors and metastases within one patient.[22,23] Intratumoral heterogeneity, the discordant PD-L1 expression between tumor biopsy and surgical specimen from one tumor, adds the risk of sampling error and could lead to an overestimation or underestimation of the PD-L1 status of all tumor tissue in a patient.[24] Furthermore, PD-L1 expression varies over time, in response to a constantly evolving immune response[1] and to anticancer treatment as demonstrated by the upregulation of PD-L1 after radiotherapy treatment.[25]

Second, each available validated IHC-assay uses different antibody clones, platforms, thresholds, and scoring algorithms.[26–28] The feasibility of harmonizing the clinical use of 4 commercial PD-L1 IHC assays has been studied in NSCLC, concluding that 3 of 4 assays are able to similarly detect tumor PD-L1 expression.[29,30] Nevertheless, interchanging assays and cutoffs leads to "misclassification" of PD-L1 status for 37% of patients, and this has important clinical consequences, as patients are potentially withheld from ICI treatment.[29,30]

The pitfalls in the IHC analysis of PD-L1 have boosted the development of new tumor tissue, blood-based, and imaging biomarker research

strategies (**Table 1**). Examples are multiplex IHC that allows for simultaneous quantification of multiple immune checkpoint molecules differentially expressed on immune and tumor cells.[31,32] Furthermore, the assessment of PD-L1 using next-generation sequencing (NGS) has shown comparable results to PD-L1 IHC analyses[33] and blood-based biomarkers such as PD-1+ CD8+ T cells have been associated with response to PD-1 targeting ICI.[34,35] Also, PD-L1 expressing circulating tumor cells showed a good correlation with tumor PD-L1 and might serve as a predictor of early response to ICI targeting PD-1.[36,37]

Molecular imaging modalities can function as a complementary tool to guide the development of effective ICI treatment strategies.[38] Using radiolabeled tracers, molecular imaging allows noninvasive visualization of all accessible PD-1/PD-L1,[39–43] including its heterogeneous expression across metastases on a whole-body level. This approach also suits the dynamic nature of PD-L1/PD-1, as it reflects the actual PD-L1/PD-1 status instead of a historical PD-L1/PD-1 status that may have been subject to change. Repetitive imaging enables on-treatment assessment of PD-L1 expression and provides a unique insight into the therapy-induced changes[44] and might support alternative treatment planning (eg, radiotherapy before ICI in low PD-L1 expression tumor

Table 1
Summary of the characteristics of the currently explored biomarkers to visualize PD-1/PD-L1

Ideal PD-1/ PD-L1 Biomarker Features	IHC	Flow cytometry[a]	NGS[b]	PD-1/ PD-L1 PET
Noninvasive	-	√√	-	√√
Cheap	√√	√	-	-
Fast	√	√	√	-
Longitudinal/ dynamic	-	√√	-	√√
Whole-body	-	-	-	√√
Applicable in clinic/as standard	√√	√√	√	√
Quantification	√	√	√	√
Sensitivity	√	√	√	√√

Abbreviations: IHC, immunohistochemistry; NGS, next-generation sequencing; PD-1/PD-L1, programmed cell death-1/programmed cell death ligand-1; √√, yes; √, moderate; -, no.
[a] Blood based.
[b] Tumor tissue based.

lesions). Finally, it allows for a better understanding of the in vivo distribution and behavior of targeted drugs; for example, drug delivery over time, drug dynamics related to dosing[39,45]

In Vivo Molecular Imaging

In vivo molecular imaging requires radiolabeling of a compound of interest using a radionuclide that matches the compounds size and half-life, followed by visualization with Single Photon Emission computed tomography (SPECT) or PET imaging.[45] We describe the current status of preclinical and clinical PD-1/PD-L1 imaging studies, and discuss major challenges in analyzing and interpreting their results.

Preclinical programmed cell death-1/ programmed cell death ligand-1 imaging studies

Several preclinical studies have demonstrated the feasibility of radionuclide imaging to noninvasively assess PD-1/PD-L1 expression. In preclinical studies, tracers can be directed against human PD-1/PD-L1 to validate tracers for subsequent clinical use. These tracers are evaluated in immune deficient mice bearing human xenografts or in humanized mice models; mice transplanted with human immune cells. Other tracers are directed against murine PD-1/PD-L1 to investigate the distribution of these agents in animals with a fully functioning immune system. Both strategies have provided valuable information about the potential role of PD-1/PD-L1 imaging to better understand and predict the efficacy of ICI.

Different tracer molecules have been developed to image PD-L1 and PD-1. Radiolabeled PD-L1 antibodies can distinguish tumors with different PD-L1 expression levels and allow for monitoring of therapy-induced changes in PD-L1 expression in preclinical tumor models.[42–44,46] For example, Hettich and colleagues[43] developed a copper-64 (^{64}Cu) labeled anti-mouse PD-1 antibody to image PD-1 positive cells in murine tumor models, demonstrating specific tracer uptake in lymphoid organs (lymph nodes and spleen). In the same model, ^{64}Cu-labeled anti-PD-1 PET was able to measure the infiltration of PD-1 positive cells in melanoma lesions in mice that were treated with a combination of radiotherapy and CTLA-4/PD-L1 inhibitors, suggesting that PD-1 PET might be used for ICI treatment monitoring.

In another study, the clinically approved PD-1 inhibitor pembrolizumab labeled with zirconium-89 (^{89}Zr) was evaluated, demonstrating its potential to image tumor infiltration of adoptively transferred human peripheral blood mononuclear cells in humanized mice engrafted with melanoma tumors.[47] Next to these studies, several other radiolabeled antibodies, nanobodies, and affibody molecules have preclinically demonstrated to be excellent tracers for noninvasive imaging of PD-L1 and PD-1.[41,48,49]

Clinical programmed cell death-1/programmed cell death ligand-1 imaging studies

Most clinical PD-1/PD-L1 imaging studies use ^{89}Zr-labeled monoclonal antibodies, which combine the sensitivity of PET with the specificity of the antibody, resulting in whole-body PET imaging in a sensitive and quantitative manner.[40,45,50,51]

Recently, Bensch and colleagues[52] reported the first clinical PD-L1 PET imaging study with ^{89}Zr-labeled anti-PD-L1 monoclonal antibody atezolizumab in 22 patients with either locally advanced or metastatic bladder cancer, NSCLC, or triple negative breast cancer. Patients received 10 mg unlabeled atezolizumab followed by ^{89}Zr-atezolizumab (37 MBq, ~1 mg antibody) intravenously. Imaging was performed at 4 and 7 days postinjection, and subsequent atezolizumab treatment was started until disease progression (Fig. 1). The investigators concluded that ^{89}Zr-atezolizumab injection was safe, apart from one grade 3 infusion-related reaction. In normal tissue, increased ^{89}Zr-atezolizumab uptake over time was observed in intestines, kidney, liver, and bone marrow. Furthermore, ^{89}Zr-atezolizumab demonstrated high but variable uptake in nonmalignant lymph nodes and spleen. The standardized uptake value (SUV)$_{max}$ ^{89}Zr-atezolizumab tumor uptake was 10.4 (95% confidence interval [CI] 8.5–12.7; range 1.6–46.1), with major intratumoral and intertumoral heterogeneity (Fig. 2). ^{89}Zr-atezolizumab tumor uptake was related to clinical response; patients with complete response had a 2.35-fold higher SUV$_{max}$ than patients with immediate progression (95% CI 98%–476%; $P<.001$).

Niemeijer and colleagues[53] published a study using the anti-PD-1 monoclonal antibody nivolumab radiolabeled with ^{89}Zr. A total of 13 patients with advanced NSCLC received ^{89}Zr-nivolumab (37 MBq ± 10%, 2 mg antibody) followed by PET/computed tomography at 162 hours (~7 days) postinjection. Subsequently, nivolumab treatment was initiated. The tracer injection was considered safe in the absence of grade ≥3 tracer-related adverse events. Quantitative PET-analyses revealed high tracer accumulation in spleen and liver. ^{89}Zr-nivolumab tumor uptake was higher in patients with immunohistochemically proven PD-1 positive tumor-infiltrating immune cells as compared with PD-1 negative tumors (median SUV$_{peak}$ 7.0 vs 2.7, P = .03).

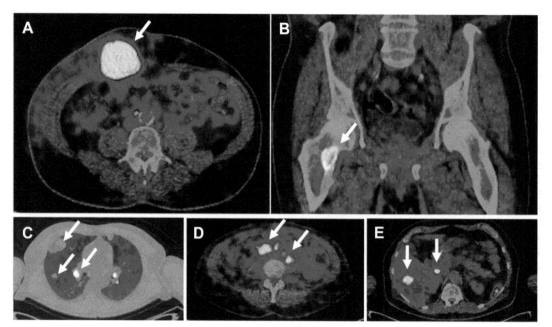

Fig. 1. Examples of PET/CT images of 4 patients illustrating [89]Zr-atezolizumab tumor uptake in 5 different locations on day 7 postinjection (*white arrows* indicate tumor lesions; PET scans were performed once per patient and time point). Images (*A*) and (*B*) are from the same patient, whereas images (*C*), (*D*), and (*E*) are from a separate patient each. (*From* Bensch F, van der Veen EL, Lub-de Hooge MN, et al. (89)Zr-atezolizumab imaging as a non-invasive approach to assess clinical response to PD-L1 blockade in cancer. Nature medicine. 2018;24(12):1852-1858[53], with permission.)

[89]Zr-nivolumab uptake did not correlate with high tumor PD-L1 expression. Visual [89]Zr-nivolumab tumor uptake revealed significant heterogeneity, both between and within patients. [89]Zr-nivolumab tumor uptake was related to clinical response; of lesions with a diameter of $\geq$20 mm, the SUV_{peak} was numerically higher in responding lesions compared with nonresponding lesions (median SUV_{peak} 6.4 vs 3.0, P = .019).

In addition to the first clinical studies with radiolabeled PD-1/PD-L1 monoclonal antibodies, Xing and colleagues[54] were the first to demonstrate clinical single-domain antibodies (sdAbs) or nanobody SPECT-imaging. They reported results from 16 patients with advanced NSCLC using NM-01 (anti-PD-L1), which was radiolabeled site-specifically with [99m]Tc. The administered dose of 3.8 to 10.4 MBq/kg, corresponding to 100 or 400 μg of NM-01, was considered to be safe. SPECT scans were acquired at 1 and 2 hours postinjection, resulting in visible tumor uptake at 2 hours postinjection. Average tumor to blood

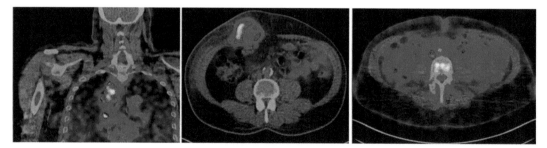

Fig. 2. PET/CT images of lesions of 3 patients with heterogeneous [89]Zr-atezolizumab uptake between lesions on day 7 postinjection (PET scans were performed once per patient and time point). Mediastinal lesion of a patient with NSCLC (SUV_{max} 19.9) (*left*), an abdominal wall metastases of a patient with bladder cancer (SUV_{max} 36.4) (*middle*), and a bone metastasis of a patient with triple negative breast cancer (SUV_{max} 7.1) (*right*). (*From*: Bensch F, van der Veen EL, Lub-de Hooge MN, et al. (89)Zr-atezolizumab imaging as a non-invasive approach to assess clinical response to PD-L1 blockade in cancer. Nature medicine. 2018;24(12):1852-1858[53], with permission.)

pool ratios (T:BP) at 2 hours varied from 1.24 to 3.53 and correlated well with PD-L1 expression measured immunohistochemically. Visual intratumoral and intertumoral heterogeneity of tracer uptake was noted in some primary tumors and among several patients. Patients with a PD-L1 expression ≤1% tend to show a lower T:BP radio (mean 1.89 vs 2.49, P = .048).

Finally, Niemeijer and colleagues[53] reported clinical PET imaging data with ^{18}F-anti-PD-L1 adnectin (BMS-986192) in patients with advanced NSCLC. Patients received 3 MBq/kg ^{18}F-BMS-986192 (specific activity ≥6.1 GBq/μmol) and a PET scan was acquired at 1 hour postinjection. SUV_{peak} for lesions with ≥50% tumor PD-L1 expression was significantly higher compared with lesions with less than 50% tumor PD-L1 expression, according to IHC (8.2 vs 2.9, P = .018). Visual ^{18}F-BMS-986192 uptake heterogeneity was observed both between and within patients. Again, SUV_{peak} for responding lesions was higher than nonresponding lesions (median 6.5 vs 3.2, P = .03).

Limitations and Challenges of Programmed Cell Death-1/Programmed Cell Death Ligand-1 Imaging

Currently, multiple clinical PD-1/L1 imaging studies are awaited or ongoing (**Table 2**). Their main hypothesis is that PD-1/PD-L1 imaging will enable us to (1) study the tumor and normal tissue targeting of PD-1/L1 ICI, (2) determine the correlation between PD-1/PD-L1 targeting of various metastases and their response to ICI, (3) understand the mechanism of action of ICI, and (4) assess the dynamics of PD-L1/PD-1 on anticancer treatment. First clinical studies have demonstrated that PD-1/PD-L1 imaging using radiolabeled antibodies, small peptides or sdAbs is feasible and safe. Their results suggest a relation between tracer uptake and IHC PD-L1 expression, as well as a relation between tracer uptake and ICI response. However, they were conducted in a limited number of patients and besides technical limitations, the correct interpretation of tracer uptake is challenging and various contributing factors should be taken into account.

Table 2
Ongoing and awaited clinical PD-1/PD-L1 imaging studies

Clinical Trial	Phase	Imaging Technique	Tumor Type	Patients, n
2015-004760-11	Completed	[^{18}F]F-PD-L1 PET and [^{89}Zr]Zr-nivolumab PET	NSCLC	10
NCT02453984	Completed	[^{89}Zr]Zr-atezolizumab PET	Locally advanced or metastatic solid tumors	22
NCT03514719 (PINNACLE)	Recruiting	[^{89}Zr]Zr-avelumab PET	NSCLC	37
NCT03829007 (PINCH)	Recruiting	[^{89}Zr]Zr-durvalumab PET and [^{18}F]F-FDG PET	HNSCC	58
2015-005765-23	Recruiting	[^{89}Zr]Zr-durvalumab PET	NSCLC	10
NCT03520634	unknown	[^{18}F]F-PD-L1 PET	Melanoma	15
NCT02760225	Active, not recruiting	[^{89}Zr]Zr-pembrolizumab PET	Melanoma/NSCLC	18
NCT03065764	Active, not recruiting	[^{89}Zr]Zr-pembrolizumab PET	NSCLC	10
NCT03843515 (NeoNivo)	Recruiting	[^{18}F]F-FDG PET and [^{18}F]F-PD-L1 PET	Oral cavity squamous cell carcinoma	15
NCT02978196	Recruiting	[^{99m}Tc]Tc-anti-PD-L1 (sdAb) SPECT	NSCLC	50
NCT03850028	Not yet recruiting	[^{89}Zr]Zr-atezolizumab PET	DLBCL	20
NCT03853187 (DONAN)	Recruiting	[^{89}Zr]Zr-durvalumab PET and [^{111}In]In- CD8 T-cell SPECT	NSCLC	20

Abbreviations: DLBCL, diffuse large B-cell lymphoma; [^{18}F]F-FDG PET, PET with fludeoxyglucose F 18; NSCLC, non–small-cell lung cancer; PD-1/PD-L1, programmed cell death-1/programmed cell death ligand-1; sdAb, single-domain antibody; ^{89}Zr, zirconium 89.

For example, the image quality of PET imaging is limited by the low spatial resolution that results in a partial volume effect mainly affecting small and low-contrast tumor lesions. Also, measurement errors can occur due to a low signal-to-noise ratio, caused by low injected activity doses and the low positron abundance of [89]Zr.[55] Therefore, heterogenic tracer uptake should be interpreted with caution in the absence of histologic confirmation of target expression, as visual variable uptake may not reflect true heterogenic PD-L1 expression but noise-induced variability of the quantitative target-uptake measurements as previously described by Jauw and colleagues.[55] Variable tracer uptake may also result from differences in perfusion and accessibility in tumor and normal tissues.[56] Thus, it could be that PD-1/PD-L1 expression is present, but due to limited perfusion, the radiolabeled antibody is not able to reach its target.

Third, knowledge on the target expression levels is not only essential to accurately interpret the acquired scan, but also to find optimal dosing levels for imaging. Immune cells in the spleen often express PD-L1 because of their physiologic role in regulating the immune response. Therefore, the spleen acts as a sink organ for PD-L1 radiotracers. At low antibody doses, most of the injected tracer will accumulate in the spleen, resulting in rapid blood clearance and minimal targeting to other PD-L1–positive tissues like the tumor.[44,57] By increasing the antibody dose, spleen uptake saturates, resulting in restored circulation time and increased targeting to tumor and other PD-L1–positive tissue.[52] Contrary to PD-L1, expression levels of PD-1 on immune cells are much lower and there is no sink organ affecting the biodistribution of PD-1 targeting tracers. Therefore, lower doses should be used to prevent saturation of all PD-1 and to obtain high-contrast images.[43,53]

The physiologic presence of PD-1/PD-L1 in various types of cells (eg, tumor, immune, or other cell types), challenges the interpretation of visual tracer uptake.[43,44,57] Histologic confirmation is therefore advisable and, for example, multiplex IHC could be used for the identification of each cell type, taken all previously mentioned limitations of IHC on tumor biopsies into account. The addition of another imaging technique (eg, PET with fludeoxyglucose F 18) is also worth considering to distinguish between physiologic targeting from receptor-mediated targeting, or identify different cell types. However, this remains extremely challenging.

Finally, knowledge of the (differences in) makeup of currently available antibodies targeting PD-1/PD-L1 is essential for correct interpretation of (variable) tracer uptake.[58] Especially the interaction between the Fc-region of the antibody with the Fc-gamma receptors (FcγRs) presenting immunoglobulin (Ig)G subtypes. Vivier and colleagues[59] suggested that the binding of humanized IgG1 by FcγRI contributes to the uptake of radiolabeled immuno-conjugates in nontarget tissues during antibody-based PET imaging. Based on their findings, the use of deglycosylated radiolabeled immuno-conjugates is proposed to decrease unwanted uptake in healthy organs, thereby optimizing the imaging quality and interpretation.

FUTURE PERSPECTIVES

The prospect of ICI treatment strategies lies in our ability to translate our increasing understanding of the human immune responses in the tumor microenvironment to more effective treatments. PD-L1 assessment on tumor biopsies using IHC is unlikely to play a role in this respect.[2,3] PD-1/PD-L1 imaging has shown to visualize whole-body PD-1/PD-L1 expression and accessibility. However, the presence of single immune checkpoints is likely an oversimplification of factors determining ICI therapy response. Therefore, PD-1/PD-L1 imaging may give a more accurate representation of whole-body PD-1/PD-L1 expression compared with IHC PD-L1, but its role as predictor of response remains to be determined. Next to pretreatment imaging, it would be very relevant to explore the feasibility of (repetitive) on-treatment imaging to assess the dynamics of PD-L1/PD-1 on anticancer treatment.

Different types of radiotracers have already demonstrated their potential in the (pre)clinical setting to image PD-1/PD-L1, including intact monoclonal antibodies, nanobodies, and adnectins. Which one is most suitable depends on the research question. For example, smaller proteins, such as nanobodies and peptides, can be of growing interest because they are rapidly eliminated from the bloodstream and can reach the core of tumors, whereas antibodies may be more limited in their tissue-penetrating capacity because of their size.[48] Therefore, these molecules may be more suitable to answer fundamental research questions about the expression levels of immune checkpoints in tumors. On the other hand, intact therapeutic antibodies provide us with important information of the whole-body distribution of ICI and the accessibility of tumors for monoclonal antibodies in the clinical setting.

In addition to PD-1/PD-L1 imaging, further insights into the fundamental mechanisms that regulate early aspects of T-cell activation will provide key information to better understand the variable ICI response rates. In this respect, some promising molecular imaging approaches have been reported recently.[16,60–62] Imaging CD8+ T cells using antibody fragments allows for direct assessment of the location, density, and proximity of CD8+ T cells, which is relevant because ICI invigorates CD8+ T-cell responses to specific tumor antigens.[63,64] Several clinical studies in lymphoma and solid malignancies (NCT03802123, NCT03610061) are ongoing; however, a tolerogenic tumor microenvironment can inhibit the activity of cytotoxic T cells. Granzyme B is a serine-protease released from CD8+ T cells and natural killer cells, and is one of the key markers for immune cell activation. Granzyme B PET imaging using a targeted peptide, GZP, can visualize and quantify granzyme B; therefore, it allows for the identification of active tumor infiltrating lymphocytes to monitor the therapeutic efficacy of ICI treatment.[65] Currently, the in vivo visualization of active TILs is being evaluated using [^{18}F]F-AraG PET/MR in patients with urothelial carcinoma receiving neo-adjuvant anti-PD-1/PD-L1 ICI treatment (NCT03007719).

SUMMARY

The rapidly evolving landscape of immune-oncology is promising, but also leaves many yet unanswered questions. Recent clinical studies have demonstrated feasibility of PD-1/PD-L1 imaging to visualize PD-L/PD-L1 expression in clinical studies. These emerging noninvasive, whole-body and quantitative tools serve to improve our understanding of the dynamic tumor microenvironment and enable optimization of ICI-based strategies.

REFERENCES

1. Sharma P, Allison JP. The future of immune checkpoint therapy. Science 2015;348(6230):56–61.
2. Reck M, Rodriguez-Abreu D, Robinson AG, et al. Pembrolizumab versus chemotherapy for PD-L1-positive non-small-cell lung cancer. N Engl J Med 2016;375(19):1823–33.
3. Rittmeyer A, Barlesi F, Waterkamp D, et al. Atezolizumab versus docetaxel in patients with previously treated non-small-cell lung cancer (OAK): a phase 3, open-label, multicentre randomised controlled trial. Lancet 2017;389(10066):255–65.
4. Cohen EEW, Soulières D, Le Tourneau C, et al. Pembrolizumab versus methotrexate, docetaxel, or cetuximab for recurrent or metastatic head-and-neck squamous cell carcinoma (KEYNOTE-040): a randomised, open-label, phase 3 study. Lancet 2019; 393(10167):156–67.
5. Weber JS, Mandalà M, Vecchio MD, et al. Adjuvant therapy with nivolumab (NIVO) versus ipilimumab (IPI) after complete resection of stage III/IV melanoma: updated results from a phase III trial (CheckMate 238). J Clin Oncol 2018;36(15_suppl):9502.
6. Postow MA, Chesney J, Pavlick AC, et al. Nivolumab and ipilimumab versus ipilimumab in untreated melanoma. N Engl J Med 2015;372(21):2006–17.
7. Harrington KJ, Ferris RL, Blumenschein G, et al. Nivolumab versus standard, single-agent therapy of investigator's choice in recurrent or metastatic squamous cell carcinoma of the head and neck (CheckMate 141): health-related quality-of-life results from a randomised, phase 3 trial. Lancet Oncol 2017; 18(8):1104–15.
8. Gaiser MR, Bongiorno M, Brownell I. PD-L1 inhibition with avelumab for metastatic Merkel cell carcinoma. Expert Rev Clin Pharmacol 2018;11(4): 345–59.
9. Motzer RJ, Tannir NM, McDermott DF, et al. Nivolumab plus ipilimumab versus sunitinib in advanced renal-cell carcinoma. N Engl J Med 2018;378(14): 1277–90.
10. Bellmunt J, de Wit R, Vaughn DJ, et al. Pembrolizumab as second-line therapy for advanced urothelial carcinoma. N Engl J Med 2017;376(11):1015–26.
11. Hargadon KM, Johnson CE, Williams CJ. Immune checkpoint blockade therapy for cancer: an overview of FDA-approved immune checkpoint inhibitors. Int Immunopharmacol 2018;62:29–39.
12. Sanmamed MF, Chen L. A paradigm shift in cancer immunotherapy: from enhancement to normalization. Cell 2018;175(2):313–26.
13. Antonia SJ, Villegas A, Daniel D, et al. Overall survival with durvalumab after chemoradiotherapy in stage III NSCLC. N Engl J Med 2018;379(24): 2342–50.
14. Fridman WH, Pagès F, Sautès-Fridman C, et al. The immune contexture in human tumours: impact on clinical outcome. Nat Rev Cancer 2012;12:298.
15. Chen DS, Mellman I. Elements of cancer immunity and the cancer-immune set point. Nature 2017; 541(7637):321–30.
16. Tumeh PC, Harview CL, Yearley JH, et al. PD-1 blockade induces responses by inhibiting adaptive immune resistance. Nature 2014;515(7528): 568–71.
17. Hamid O, Robert C, Daud A, et al. Safety and tumor responses with lambrolizumab (anti-PD-1) in melanoma. N Engl J Med 2013;369(2):134–44.
18. Binnewies M, Roberts EW, Kersten K, et al. Understanding the tumor immune microenvironment (TIME) for effective therapy. Nat Med 2018;24(5): 541–50.
19. Tang J, Shalabi A, Hubbard-Lucey VM. Comprehensive analysis of the clinical immuno-oncology landscape. Ann Oncol 2018;29(1):84–91.

20. Fruhwirth GO, Kneilling M, de Vries IJM, et al. The potential of in vivo imaging for optimization of molecular and cellular anti-cancer immunotherapies. Mol Imaging Biol 2018;20(5):696–704.

21. Hofman P. The challenges of evaluating predictive biomarkers using small biopsy tissue samples and liquid biopsies from non-small cell lung cancer patients. J Thorac Dis 2019;11(Suppl 1):S57–s64.

22. Kluger HM, Zito CR, Turcu G, et al. PD-L1 studies across tumor types, its differential expression and predictive value in patients treated with immune checkpoint inhibitors. Clin Cancer Res 2017; 23(15):4270–9.

23. Madore J, Vilain RE, Menzies AM, et al. PD-L1 expression in melanoma shows marked heterogeneity within and between patients: implications for anti-PD-1/PD-L1 clinical trials. Pigment Cell Melanoma Res 2015;28(3):245–53.

24. Ilie M, Long-Mira E, Bence C, et al. Comparative study of the PD-L1 status between surgically resected specimens and matched biopsies of NSCLC patients reveal major discordances: a potential issue for anti-PD-L1 therapeutic strategies. Ann Oncol 2016;27(1):147–53.

25. Twyman-Saint Victor C, Rech AJ, Maity A, et al. Radiation and dual checkpoint blockade activate nonredundant immune mechanisms in cancer. Nature 2015;520(7547):373–7.

26. Udall M, Rizzo M, Kenny J, et al. PD-L1 diagnostic tests: a systematic literature review of scoring algorithms and test-validation metrics. Diagn Pathol 2018;13(1):12.

27. Algenas C, Agaton C, Fagerberg L, et al. Antibody performance in western blot applications is context-dependent. Biotechnol J 2014;9(3):435–45.

28. Mathew M, Safyan RA, Shu CA. PD-L1 as a biomarker in NSCLC: challenges and future directions. Ann Transl Med 2017;5(18):375.

29. Hirsch FR, McElhinny A, Stanforth D, et al. PD-L1 immunohistochemistry assays for lung cancer: results from phase 1 of the blueprint PD-L1 IHC assay comparison project. J Thorac Oncol 2017;12(2): 208–22.

30. Tsao MS, Kerr KM, Kockx M, et al. PD-L1 immunohistochemistry comparability study in real-life clinical samples: results of blueprint phase 2 project. J Thorac Oncol 2018;13(9):1302–11.

31. Stack EC, Foukas PG, Lee PP. Multiplexed tissue biomarker imaging. J Immunother Cancer 2016;4:9.

32. Gorris MAJ, Halilovic A, Rabold K, et al. Eight-color multiplex immunohistochemistry for simultaneous detection of multiple immune checkpoint molecules within the tumor microenvironment. J Immunol 2018;200(1):347–54.

33. Conroy JM, Pabla S, Nesline MK, et al. Next generation sequencing of PD-L1 for predicting response to immune checkpoint inhibitors. J Immunother Cancer 2019;7(1):18.

34. Zelba H, Bochem J, Pawelec G, et al. Accurate quantification of T-cells expressing PD-1 in patients on anti-PD-1 immunotherapy. Cancer Immunol Immunother 2018;67(12):1845–51.

35. Gros A, Robbins PF, Yao X, et al. PD-1 identifies the patient-specific CD8(+) tumor-reactive repertoire infiltrating human tumors. J Clin Invest 2014; 124(5):2246–59.

36. Yue C, Jiang Y, Li P, et al. Dynamic change of PD-L1 expression on circulating tumor cells in advanced solid tumor patients undergoing PD-1 blockade therapy. Oncoimmunology 2018;7(7): e1438111.

37. Ilié M, Szafer-Glusman E, Hofman V, et al. Detection of PD-L1 in circulating tumor cells and white blood cells from patients with advanced non-small-cell lung cancer. Ann Oncol 2017;29(1):193–9.

38. Cohen JV, Flaherty KT. Response to immune checkpoint antibodies: not all responses are created equal. Clin Cancer Res 2019;25(3):910–1.

39. Lamberts LE, Williams SP, Terwisscha van Scheltinga AG, et al. Antibody positron emission tomography imaging in anticancer drug development. J Clin Oncol 2015;33(13):1491–504.

40. Jauw YW, Menke-van der Houven van Oordt CW, Hoekstra OS, et al. Immuno-positron emission tomography with zirconium-89-labeled monoclonal antibodies in oncology: what can we learn from initial clinical trials? Front Pharmacol 2016;7:131.

41. Broos K, Keyaerts M, Lecocq Q, et al. Non-invasive assessment of murine PD-L1 levels in syngeneic tumor models by nuclear imaging with nanobody tracers. Oncotarget 2017;8(26):41932–46.

42. Heskamp S, Hobo W, Molkenboer-Kuenen JD, et al. Noninvasive imaging of tumor PD-L1 expression using radiolabeled anti-PD-L1 antibodies. Cancer Res 2015;75(14):2928–36.

43. Hettich M, Braun F, Bartholoma MD, et al. High-resolution PET imaging with therapeutic antibody-based PD-1/PD-L1 checkpoint tracers. Theranostics 2016;6(10):1629–40.

44. Heskamp S, Wierstra PJ, Molkenboer-Kuenen JDM, et al. PD-L1 microSPECT/CT imaging for longitudinal monitoring of PD-L1 expression in syngeneic and humanized mouse models for cancer. Cancer Immunol Res 2019;7(1):150–61.

45. Waaijer SJH, Kok IC, Eisses B, et al. Molecular imaging in cancer drug development. J Nucl Med 2018; 59(5):726–32.

46. Kikuchi M, Clump DA, Srivastava RM, et al. Preclinical immunoPET/CT imaging using Zr-89-labeled anti-PD-L1 monoclonal antibody for assessing radiation-induced PD-L1 upregulation in head and neck cancer and melanoma. Oncoimmunology 2017;6(7):e1329071.

47. Natarajan A, Mayer AT, Reeves RE, et al. Development of Novel ImmunoPET tracers to image human PD-1 checkpoint expression on tumor-infiltrating lymphocytes in a humanized mouse model. Mol Imaging Biol 2017;19(6):903–14.

48. Broos K, Lecocq Q, Raes G, et al. Noninvasive imaging of the PD-1:PD-L1 immune checkpoint: embracing nuclear medicine for the benefit of personalized immunotherapy. Theranostics 2018; 8(13):3559–70.

49. Gonzalez Trotter DE, Meng X, McQuade P, et al. In vivo imaging of the programmed death ligand 1 by (18)F PET. J Nucl Med 2017;58(11):1852–7.

50. Wu AM, Olafsen T. Antibodies for molecular imaging of cancer. Cancer J 2008;14(3):191–7.

51. Van Dongen GA, Huisman MC, Boellaard R, et al. 89Zr-immuno-PET for imaging of long circulating drugs and disease targets: why, how and when to be applied? Q J Nucl Med Mol Imaging 2015; 59(1):18–38.

52. Bensch F, van der Veen EL, Lub-de Hooge MN, et al. (89)Zr-atezolizumab imaging as a non-invasive approach to assess clinical response to PD-L1 blockade in cancer. Nat Med 2018;24(12):1852–8.

53. Niemeijer AN, Leung D, Huisman MC, et al. Whole body PD-1 and PD-L1 positron emission tomography in patients with non-small-cell lung cancer. Nat Commun 2018;9(1):4664.

54. Xing Y, Chand G, Liu C, et al. Early phase I study of a (99m)Tc labeled anti-PD-L1 single domain antibody in SPECT/CT assessment of programmed death ligand-1 expression in non-small cell lung cancer. J Nucl Med 2019;60(9):1213–20.

55. Jauw YWS, Heijtel DF, Zijlstra JM, et al. Noise-induced variability of immuno-PET with zirconium-89-labeled antibodies: an analysis based on count-reduced clinical images. Mol Imaging Biol 2018;20(6):1025–34.

56. Oosting SF, Brouwers AH, van Es SC, et al. 89Zr-bevacizumab PET visualizes heterogeneous tracer accumulation in tumor lesions of renal cell carcinoma patients and differential effects of antiangiogenic treatment. J Nucl Med 2015;56(1):63–9.

57. Nedrow JR, Josefsson A, Park S, et al. Imaging of programmed cell death ligand 1: impact of protein concentration on distribution of anti-PD-L1 SPECT agents in an immunocompetent murine model of melanoma. J Nucl Med 2017;58(10):1560–6.

58. Arce Vargas F, Furness AJS, Litchfield K, et al. Fc effector function contributes to the activity of human anti-CTLA-4 antibodies. Cancer cell 2018;33(4): 649–63.e4.

59. Vivier D, Sharma SK, Adumeau P, et al. The impact of FcgammaRI binding on ImmunoPET. J Nucl Med 2019;60(8):1174–82.

60. Herbst RS, Soria JC, Kowanetz M, et al. Predictive correlates of response to the anti-PD-L1 antibody MPDL3280A in cancer patients. Nature 2014; 515(7528):563–7.

61. Powles T, Eder JP, Fine GD, et al. MPDL3280A (anti-PD-L1) treatment leads to clinical activity in metastatic bladder cancer. Nature 2014;515(7528):558–62.

62. Ratcliffe MJ, Sharpe A, Midha A, et al. Agreement between programmed cell death ligand-1 diagnostic assays across multiple protein expression cutoffs in non-small cell lung cancer. Clin Cancer Res 2017;23(14):3585–91.

63. Slaney CY, Kershaw MH, Darcy PK. Trafficking of T cells into tumors. Cancer Res 2014;74(24):7168–74.

64. Bellone M, Calcinotto A. Ways to enhance lymphocyte trafficking into tumors and fitness of tumor infiltrating lymphocytes. Front Oncol 2013;3:231.

65. Larimer BM, Bloch E, Nesti S, et al. The effectiveness of checkpoint inhibitor combinations and administration timing can Be measured by granzyme B PET imaging. Clin Cancer Res 2019;25(4): 1196–205.

The Role of Positron Emission Tomography Imaging in Radiotherapy Target Delineation

Hari Menon, BS[a], Chunxiao Guo, MD[b], Vivek Verma, MD[c],
Charles B. Simone II, MD[d],*

KEYWORDS

• PET imaging • Radiation oncology • Target delineation • Treatment planning • Target volume

KEY POINTS

- Positron emission tomography (PET) can offer considerable advantages for target volume delineation as part of radiation treatment planning.
- Examples from 6 general oncology disease sites are assessed in this review to descriptively evaluate the role of PET in target volume delineation.
- Specific utilities include differentiating tumor from normal tissue as well as initial target volume delineation and radiotherapy delivery.
- Exploratory utilities include focal radiation dose escalation, adaptive treatment planning, and treatment optimization by risk status.

INTRODUCTION

Until relatively recently, the ability to diagnose and treat cancer with radiation therapy (RT) has been largely based on anatomy, without consideration of metabolic or dynamic capabilities. Computed tomography (CT) and magnetic resonance imaging (MRI) are advanced imaging modalities that can use differences in Hounsfield units, density, contrast uptake, and other features to identify malignant structures versus normal tissues. In contrast, positron emission tomography (PET), a form of functional imaging, has become an indispensable tool for oncologic diagnosis, staging, prognostication, and surveillance.

This use of PET imaging can be directly applied to radiation oncology and radiation target delineation.[1] Currently, virtually all radiation treatment planning systems utilize CT and/or MRI-based target delineation, but PET imaging is increasingly being integrated within RT planning. This review highlights and summarizes current literature regarding the use of PET imaging in the setting of RT target delineation (**Box 1**).

CENTRAL NERVOUS SYSTEM

Brain imaging has not typically utilized [18F]-fluorodeoxyglucose (FDG) PET owing to its relatively limited differentiation and sensitivity due to the

Funding: There were no funding sources for this work.
Disclosures: All authors declare that conflicts of interest do not exist.
[a] University of Arizona College of Medicine, 475 N 5th St, Phoenix, AZ 85004, USA; [b] Department of Interventional Radiology, University of Texas MD Anderson Cancer Center, 1515 Holcombe Blvd, Houston, TX 77030, USA; [c] Department of Radiation Oncology, Allegheny General Hospital, 320 E North Ave, Pittsburgh, PA 15212, USA; [d] Department of Radiation Oncology, New York Proton Center, 225 East 126th Street, New York, NY 10035, USA
* Corresponding author.
E-mail address: csimone@nyproton.com

Box 1
Utility of positron emission tomography imaging in radiation oncology

- Initial cancer diagnosis
- Staging and extent of disease evaluation
- Prognosis assessment (performed using pre-treatment and/or posttreatment PETs)
- Target volume and normal tissue contour delineation
- Verify radiation dose delivery (especially for proton therapy)
- Surveillance to monitor treatment response and/or assess for recurrences
- Predict or assess for radiation-induced toxicities

---

high background uptake by normal brain tissue. FDG-PET may have utility, however, when technical and logistical modifications in technique or sequence are applied and/or when it is combined with other imaging modalities, such as MRI.[2] Hypothesis-generating studies have evaluated FDG-PET for diagnosis, prognostication, and assessment of treatment response.[3–6] Although encouraging, indications for FDG-PET, particularly for radiation target volume delineation, remain largely exploratory at this time.

Instead, recent developments in amino acid tracers have led to improved evaluation of neoplasms using PET modalities and can even provide enhanced guidance for treatment in patients who are unable to undergo MRI.[7] The most thoroughly explored amino acids studied include ^{11}C-methionine (CM)-PET and ^{18}F-fluoroethyl-L-tyrosine (FET)-PET.[8,9] In the setting of high-grade gliomas (HGGs), which are known to appear heterogeneous, these tracers may allow for better evaluation for higher risk features.

One investigative therapeutic approach using these imaging modalities is to deliver higher RT doses to higher risk or more active tumor regions. This has been previously attempted in a retrospective phase II trial of 22 patients receiving 72 Gy using a simultaneous integrated boost to areas with higher-risk features on FET-PET.[10] The results for this study appeared negative, because many of the treatment failures arose from regions that were not included in the PET-guided treatment fields, suggesting that these should be used as complementary data points for planning. To assess if such an approach and imaging-based dose escalation could be of benefit in otherwise radioresistant primary brain histologies,

additional investigation is needed, and several studies are currently under way.[11]

A study from the University of Munich has also shown advantages of CM-PET compared with postoperative MRI in the setting of resected HGGs. Although HGGs usually can be adequately discerned on T2-weighted MRI, the investigators noted that CM-PET performed better in more than 50% of patients.[12] This can allow for better delineation of gross tumor postoperatively, as demonstrated by investigators in Spain in a in a small study of 15 patients with high-grade tumors and 8 with low-grade tumors.[13] Furthermore, the value of CM-PET for tumor volume delineation can been demonstrated indirectly through its prediction of recurrence after chemoradiation. Whereas all 5 of the 19 patients who had gross tumor volumes (GTVs) based on PET imaging that was not completely confined within the high-dose region experienced noncentral failures, only 2 such failures were seen in the 14 patients with adequately covered PET-based GTVs.[14]

Additionally, amino acid PET imaging may have potential in the setting of reirradiation of HGGs. This is a particular focus of an ongoing Radiation Therapy Oncology Group (RTOG) 1205 trial (NCT01730950). The goal of that study, formed on the basis of promising retrospective data,[15,16] is to identify if CM-PET–based stereotactic treatment planning can provide durable outcomes with minimal greater than or equal to grade 3 adverse events.

HEAD AND NECK

PET/CT is a standard modality used in head and neck cancers for initial evaluation of distant metastases and post-treatment evaluation[17] and has also been evaluated for target delineation in the primary setting. Treatment planning utilizing PET/CT fusion generally provides more sharply defined GTVs compared with CT or MRI delineation.[18] Furthermore, in patients who had resection, PET-based GTVs correlated more closely with gross tumor specimens compared with other imaging modalities.[19] Furthermore, the use of more conformal GTVs, as informed by PET imaging, may allow for safer dose escalation, although studies investigating this have been limited.[20] Although additional margins are added to GTVs in radiation oncology to address microscopic tumor spread and set-up variations, more accurate GTVs and more conformal margins may reduce the irradiation exposure to adjacent critical structures, thus possibly lowering toxicities. Additionally, the utility of PET to perform adaptive therapy is also appealing,[21] particularly because the incidence of radiosensitive head and neck cancers (such as human papillomavirus-positive squamous cell carcinoma) are increasing in incidence.

PET/CT also provides particular benefit for target delineation in the setting of head and neck neoplasms of unknown primary. An analysis of 16 publications between 1994 and 2003 found that PET/CT revealed the location of primary disease in 24.5% of cases that CT, MRI, and panendoscopy could not detect.[22] This scenario has substantial implications in RT treatment and practice, because otherwise unidentified primaries can lead to larger tumor volumes receiving high irradiation doses due to the uncertainty in disease localization.

THORACIC

Non–small cell lung cancer (NSCLC) extensively utilizes PET/CT imaging for both pretreatment planning and follow-up. PET/CT fusion in this setting provides more accurate detection of metastasis compared with traditional CT modalities.[23,24] Its use in target delineation for locally advanced NSCLC[25] (and applied to limited-stage small cell lung cancer[26]) is highlighted in this text, although evidence is more limited for early-stage NSCLC.[27]

The increased sensitivity of PET/CT for nodal metastatic evaluation has augmented the lack of necessity for elective nodal irradiation.[28,29] Additionally, PET/CT-derived tumor volume definition allows for adequate dosage for areas that could otherwise be inadequately treated based on CT-imaging alone.[30] PET/CT scans can result in significant upstaging in more than half of all locally advanced NSCLC patients.[31] Similarly, PET/CT volumes also correlate more accurately with surgical specimens.[32] Lastly, PET/CT allows for better differentiation between tumor and benign lung abnormalities, such as atelectasis, which at times (along with effusions and pneumonia) can make radiation treatment planning difficult with CT-based guidance alone.[33] Similarly, lung fibrosis can commonly obscure treatment planning in the setting of reirradiation, and such patients often are better planned with PET/CT.[34–36]

Because local control continues to be problematic in locally advanced NSCLC, PET/CT in this setting may allow for focal dose escalation, as seen in several prospective trials. One such study explored a simultaneous integrated boost to areas of high FDG avidity. In 13 patients treated with this modality, 2 local failures were observed with a median follow-up of 26 months, with appropriate toxicities given the cumulative dose of 120 Gy.[37]

Such an approach was also applied in another study using a sequential stereotactic body RT (SBRT) boost to avid disease at 1 month after initial RT with moderate success.[38]

Recently, the use of PET/CT for adaptive replanning during RT for locally advanced NSCLC has become an important topic. Adaptive replanning, or modifying a treatment plan, often based on anatomic changes to the tumor volume or normal tissues during the course of radiotherapy so as to not underdose tumor or overdose normal tissues,[39] is particularly useful and often necessary when delivering RT with advanced modalities, such as proton therapy.[40] RTOG 1106, a randomized phase II study, applied adaptive planning as a therapeutic tool using PET/CT.[41] The objective for this study was to evaluate the use of interim PET/CT imaging for dose escalation (up to 86 Gy) after administration of an initial 40 Gy to 46 Gy. Interim analysis of 42 patients found appropriate in-field control with a median follow-up of 42 months. This trial was heavily influenced by several studies performed by Ding and colleagues,[42,43] who were able to safely dose-escalate after interim PET. Indiscriminate dose-escalation is still not routinely supported[44]; however, PET/CT may provide a basis for adaptive replanning by potentially allowing for safer high-dose delivery to avid areas while limiting toxicity to sensitive regions, which is particularly pertinent given the increasing recognition that cardiac dose influences overall survival (OS) in locally advanced NSCLC.[45–47]

GYNECOLOGIC

Although cervical cancer is largely staged clinically (especially in the developing world), the National Comprehensive Cancer Network (NCCN) recommends PET/CT for greater than or equal to stage 1B2 disease to guide treatment.[48] ^{18}F-FDG PET/CT imaging outperforms CT/MRI in detecting nodal disease; a recent study demonstrated that PET/CT is better able to detect para-aortic metastasis compared with CT or MRI and can allow for more informed nodal target volume delineation for radiotherapy.[49] A multicenter prospective study found that the sensitivity, specificity, positive predictive value, and negative predictive value of preoperative PET/CT were 54.8%, 97.7%, 79.3%, and 93.1%, respectively, for cervical cancer metastasis.[50]

PET/CT guided intensity-modulated RT (IMRT) was explored to treat PET-positive nodal disease by Esthappan and colleagues[51] and has been adopted at many centers despite lacking clear evidence of improved efficacy. Similarly, integrated PET/CT with MRI (or by itself) is also being studied in the setting of cervical brachyther-apy.[52,53] Snyder and colleagues[54] reported that SBRT boost (30 Gy) for PET positive lymph nodes increased tumor control probability. A recent retro-spective study also found that baseline PET imaging was associated with improved disease-specific survival.[55] In contrast, a single-center phase III trial did not demonstrate survival benefits with PET in patients receiving concurrent chemo-radiotherapy for cervical cancer and enlarged pelvic lymph nodes, but PET did detect extrapelvic metastases and did inform treatment contours by allowing for decreased use of extended-field radiotherapy.[56] Adapting PET/CT in GTV delinea-tion also reduced interobserver variation during treatment planning.[57]

Furthermore, PET imaging has been utilized to aid target definition by delineating active cervical bone marrow, because myelosuppression can impair delivery of optimal therapy in patients receiving concurrent chemoradiotherapy.[58] During treatment planning, more stringent dose limita-tions on active bone marrow can be facilitated by IMRT.[59,60] Although most studies have utilized FDG PET/CT to identify active areas of marrow proliferation, 3'-deoxy-3'-[(18)F] fluorothymidine has also been used and found comparable to FDG.[61] Zhou at al[62] showed that the absolute vol-ume of PET-defined active bone marrow spared in RT was a strong predictor of hematologic toxicity. Given the cost and availability of PET/CT imaging, a PET/CT-based atlas of active bone marrow can also assist IMRT planning for cervical cancer,[63] and PET/CT may similarly have a role in proton therapy, an emerging treatment approach for gynecologic cancers.[64]

GENITOURINARY

Due to its relatively low uptake by prostate cancer cells and urinary excretion, [18]FDG PET/CT is of more limited use for the diagnosis and treatment planning of prostate cancer.[55] Putative utilities for [18]FDG-PET in prostate cancer have been postulated for aggressive primary tumors (eg, Gleason score greater than or equal to 8), biochemical failures with negative uptake on CT imaging, and response assessment/prognostica-tion for metastatic prostate cancer.[65] The afore-mentioned indications are associated, however, with low quality and low quantity of evidence, hence cannot be recommended uniformly without more robust study.[66]

The void of [18]FDG-PET has been largely filled by many newly developed tracers. Many common isotopes, including [18]fluorine (^{18}F), [11]carbon (^{11}C), [68]gallium ([68]G), and [89]zirconium ([89]Zr), have been used to label acetate, choline, sodium fluoride, flu-ciclovine, or prostate-specific membrane antigen (PSMA). Because most tracers cannot distinguish primary prostate cancer from benign prostate hy-perplasia, studies have focused on detecting met-astatic or recurrent disease.

Both ^{18}F-labeled or ^{11}C-labeled choline have shown promise for staging of recurrent prostate cancer,[67] although the Food and Drug Administra-tion has only approved the latter to date. In a meta-analysis of 3167 patients from 47 studies, choline PET-CT had a pooled sensitivity of 0.62 and spec-ificity of 0.92 in detecting pelvic metastases.[68] Choline PET-CT also outperformed multiparamet-ric MRI in detecting nodal or bony metastases.[69] [18]F sodium fluoride (NaF) PET-CT also may prove to be a useful study for detecting bone metastases from prostate cancer. In a meta-analysis of 1170 patients from 20 studies, NaF PET-CT showed both higher sensitivity (96% vs 88%) and speci-ficity (91% vs 88%) when compared with Techne-tium methylene diphosphonate bone scintigraphy.[70] Another FDA-approved tracer is fluciclovine (anti-1-amino-3-[^{18}F] fluorocyclob utane-1-carboxylic acid), and a prospective study found superiority using it over multiparametric MRI in detecting recurrences in nonoperated patients with biochemical failure.[71] Similarly, ^{68}Ga-PSMA PET/CT performed well in detecting nodal meta-static disease and recurrence, especially when PSA levels were low.[72–75] With excellent perfor-mance in detecting nodal disease, PET/CT could have profound influence on RT, because elective nodal irradiation for intact prostate cancer is being evaluated in the randomized RTOG 0924 trial (NCT01368588).

PSMA-based PET/CT has been increasingly accepted by clinicians. A recent study by Boreta and colleagues[76] identified the locations of recur-rence after radical prostatectomy with ^{68}Ga-PSMA PET/CT. PSMA-avid disease was found in 52% of patients. This can also help inform radiation target volumes, because recurrence in 38 patients would have been inadequately treated using stan-dard salvage or nodal radiation fields. A similar study[77] in 635 biochemically recurrent patients found that the PSMA scan detection rate increased with PSA. PET-directed focal RT resulted in more than 50% reduction of PSA, implying a favorable clinical outcome. Although long-term survival and toxicity data are lacking, and the first phase 3 trial assessing the role of ^{68}Ga-PSMA PET/CT in salvage RT has just commenced,[78] these studies highlighted the potential significance of PET/CT in IMRT treatment planning. Additionally, Schwenck and colleagues[79] compared ^{68}Ga-PSMA PET/CT, ^{11}C choline PET/

CT, and CT for post-prostatectomy recurrences. They concluded that ^{68}Ga-PSMA PET/CT was the most cost-effective method to manage this patient population by avoiding incorrect treatment and providing new curative options. A similar study also found that ^{68}Ga-PSMA PET/CT was superior to ^{18}F-choline-PET/CT[80] and conventional cross-sectional imaging[81] in the detection of lymph node metastases.

The use of fluciclovine PET/CT in RT treatment planning has also been increasingly explored for RT target delineation. In a prospective study, Jani and colleagues[82] demonstrated that fluciclovine PET/CT led to a significant increase of RT target volumes without an increase in acute genitourinary or gastrointestinal toxicities. These results were echoed by another study, wherein the inclusion of fluciclovine augmented the delineation of RT target volumes in a majority of patients when compared with CT-based planning alone.[83]

LYMPHOMA

PET/CT plays an unequivocal role in management of both Hodgkin lymphoma (HL) and non-HL. Multiple consensus guidelines, as well as NCCN, recommend the use of PET/CT in the initial evaluation, treatment planning, and response assessment for these diseases.[84,85] FDG-PET/CT is also essential to modern, highly conformal RT target delineation. Current consensus guidelines have been published on recommended practices in simulation, target volume definition, and treatment planning based on PET/CT for lymphoma.[86–88]

Although PET/CT is essential for target delineation in lymphoma cases, the more emerging utility is to decide whether, based on PET/CT, targets require delineation in the first place (ie, omission of RT). This is the subject of 2 phase III trials in early-stage HL. The European Organisation for Research and Treatment of Cancer H10 Intergroup trial with 1950 patients performed interim PET/CT after 2 cycles of doxorubicin, bleomycin, vinblastine, dacarbazine (ABVD) chemotherapy; patients with a PET response (Deauville) score of 1 to 2 were randomized to involved field RT or no further treatment.[89] Noninferiority could not be demonstrated with RT omission at the end of the study: 5-year progression-free survival (PFS) rates were 99.0% in favorable patients with RT versus 87.1% without RT and 92.1% versus 89.6% in the unfavorable group. A United Kingdom trial for stage IA or IIA HL had a similar design to the H10 trial, except with 3 cycles of ABVD (n = 602) before interim PET imaging.[90] The trial showed that consolidation RT did not confer longer OS;

however, noninferiority again could not be demonstrated for 3-year PRS rates (94.6% vs 90.8%, favoring RT).

In non-HL patients, an ongoing trial is testing whether RT can be omitted in PET-negative patients after Rituximab, Cyclophosphamide, Doxorubicin Hydrochloride, Vincristine, Prednisone (R-CHOP) chemotherapy. Interim analysis found that 2-year PFS and OS rates in these patients were 79% and 88%, respectively, compared with 75% and 78%, respectively, for those who received RT in a previously published trial,[91] suggesting that avoiding RT may be acceptable in patients with negative interim PET after chemotherapy.

Given the widespread utilization of FDG PET/CT in the management of lymphoma, PET/MRI and alternative tracers are being evaluated in lymphoma patients. Ferdova and colleagues[92] reviewed hybrid PET/MRI imaging in lymphoma and found higher resolution in soft tissue. Other tracers, such as ^{18}F-fluorothymidine PET, have shown improved specificity over FDG PET in distinguishing residual lymphoma from post-treatment inflammation[93]; however, not every study has recapitulated these results.[94] A prospective cohort study demonstrated ^{68}Ga-pentixafor, a ligand for CXCR4, was superior to FDG in detecting Waldenström macroglobulinemia/lymphoplasmacytic lymphoma.[95] CM-PET was also examined in pediatric lymphoma patients and performed concordantly to FDG-PET.[96] Lastly, [89]Zr-labeled anti-CD20 antibody is being actively investigated in lymphoma patients.[97]

SUMMARY

PET imaging provides considerable advantages for radiation oncologists across several disease sites to aid in radiotherapy target volume delineation. Using instances from 6 general disease sites, this review demonstrates the use for PET imaging in differentiating tumor from normal tissue, initial target volume delineation and radiotherapy delivery, focal radiation dose escalation, adaptive treatment planning, and treatment optimization by risk status.

REFERENCES

1. Verma V, Choi JI, Sawant A, et al. Use of PET and other functional imaging to guide target delineation in radiation oncology. Semin Radiat Oncol 2018;28:171–7.
2. Kim MM, Parolia A, Dunphy MP, et al. Non-invasive metabolic imaging of brain tumours in the era of precision medicine. Nat Rev Clin Oncol 2016;13:725–39.

3. Barker FG 2nd, Chang SM, Valk PE, et al. 18-Fluoro-deoxyglucose uptake and survival of patients with suspected recurrent malignant glioma. Cancer 1997;79:115–26.

4. Delbeke D, Meyerowitz C, Lapidus RL, et al. Optimal cutoff levels of F-18 fluorodeoxyglucose uptake in the differentiation of low-grade from high-grade brain tumors with PET. Radiology 1995;195:47–52.

5. Palmedo H, Urbach H, Bender H, et al. FDG-PET in immunocompetent patients with primary central nervous system lymphoma: correlation with MRI and clinical follow-up. Eur J Nucl Med Mol Imaging 2006;33:164–8.

6. Charnley N, West CM, Barnett CM, et al. Early change in glucose metabolic rate measured using FDG-PET in patients with high-grade glioma predicts response to temozolomide but not temozolomide plus radiotherapy. Int J Radiat Oncol Biol Phys 2006;66:331–8.

7. Jaymanne DT, Kaushal S, Chan D, et al. Utilizing 18F-fluoroethyl-l-tyrosine positron emission tomography in high grade glioma for radiation treatment planning in patients with contraindications to MRI. J Med Imaging Radiat Oncol 2017;62:122–7.

8. Iuchi T, Hatano K, Uchino Y, et al. Methionine uptake and required radiation dose to control glioblastoma. Int J Radiat Oncol Biol Phys 2015;93:133–40.

9. Salber D, Stoffels G, Pauleit D, et al. Differential uptake of O-(2-18F-fluoroethyl)-L-tyrosine, L-3H-methionine, and 3H-deoxyglucose in brain abscesses. J Nucl Med 2007;48:2056–62.

10. Piroth MD, Pinkawa M, Holy R, et al. Integrated boost IMRT with FET-PET-adapted local dose escalation in glioblastomas. Results of a prospective phase II study. Strahlenther Onkol 2012;188:334–9.

11. Oehlke O, Mix M, Graf E, et al. Amino-acid PET versus MRI guided re-irradiation in patients with recurrent glioblastoma multiforme (GLIAA) – protocol of a randomized phase II trial (NOA 10/ARO 2013-1). BMC Cancer 2016;16:769.

12. Grosu AL, Weber WA, Riedel E, et al. L-(methyl-11C) methionine positron emission tomography for target delineation in resected high-grade gliomas before radiotherapy. Int J Radiat Oncol Biol Phys 2005;63:64–74.

13. Arbizu J, Tejada S, Marti-Climent JM, et al. Quantitative volumetric analysis of gliomas with sequential MRI and 11C-methionine PET assessment: patterns of integration in therapy planning. Eur J Nucl Med Mol Imaging 2012;39:771–81.

14. Lee IH, Piert M, Gomez-Hassan D, et al. Association of 11C-methionine PET uptake with site of failure after concurrent temozolomide and radiation for primary glioblastoma multiforme. Int J Radiat Oncol Biol Phys 2009;73:479–85.

15. Grosu AL, Weber WA, Franz M, et al. Reirradiation of recurrent high-grade gliomas using amino acid PET (SPECT)/CT/MRI image fusion to determine gross tumor volume for stereotactic fractionated radiotherapy. Int J Radiat Oncol Biol Phys 2005;63:511–9.

16. Miwa K, Matsuo M, Ogawa S, et al. Re-irradiation of recurrent glioblastoma multiforme using 11C-methionine PET/CT/MRI image fusion for hypofractionated stereotactic radiotherapy by intensity modulated radiation therapy. Radiat Oncol 2014;9:181.

17. Lonneux M, Hamoir M, Reychler H, et al. Positron emission tomography with [18F] fluorodeoxyglucose improves staging and patient management in patients with head and neck squamous cell carcinoma: a multicenter prospective study. J Clin Oncol 2010;28:1190–5.

18. Paulino AC, Koshy M, Howell R, et al. Comparison of CT- and FDG-PET-defined gross tumor volume in intensity-modulated radiotherapy for head-and-neck cancer. Int J Radiat Oncol Biol Phys 2005;61:1385–92.

19. Daisne JF, Duprez T, Weynand B, et al. Tumor volume in pharyngolaryngeal squamous cell carcinoma: comparison at CT, MR imaging, and FDG PET and validation with surgical specimen. Radiology 2004;233:93–100.

20. Madani I, Duthoy W, Derie C, et al. Positron emission tomography-guided, focal-dose escalation using intensity-modulated radiotherapy for head and neck cancer. Int J Radiat Oncol Biol Phys 2007;68:126–35.

21. Geets X, Tomsej M, Lee JA, et al. Adaptive biological image-guided IMRT with anatomic and functional imaging in pharyngo-laryngeal tumors: impact on target volume delineation and dose distribution using helical tomotherapy. Int J Radiat Oncol Biol Phys 2007;85:105–15.

22. Rusthoven KE, Koshy M, Paulino AC. The role of fluorodeoxyglucose positron emission tomography in cervical lymph node metastases from an unknown primary tumor. Cancer 2004;101:2641–9.

23. Pieterman RM, van Putten JW, Meuzelaar JJ, et al. Preoperative staging of non-small-cell lung cancer with positron-emission tomography. N Engl J Med 2000;343:254–61.

24. Lardinois D, Weder W, Hany TF, et al. Staging of non–small-cell lung cancer with integrated positron-emission tomography and computed tomography. N Engl J Med 2003;348:2500–7.

25. Simone CB 2nd, Houshmand S, Kalbasi A, et al. PET-based thoracic radiation oncology. PET Clin 2016;11:319–32.

26. Xanthopoulos EP, Corradetti MN, Mitra N, et al. Impact of PET staging in limited-stage small-cell lung cancer. J Thorac Oncol 2013;8:899–905.

27. Chirindel A, Adebahr S, Schuster D, et al. Impact of 4D-18FDG-PET/CT imaging on target volume delineation in SBRT patients with central versus

peripheral lung tumors. Multi-reader comparative study. Radiother Oncol 2015;115:335–41.

28. De Ruysscher D, Wanders S, van Haren E, et al. Selective mediastinal node irradiation based on FDG-PET scan data in patients with non–small-cell lung cancer: a prospective clinical study. Int J Radiat Oncol Biol Phys 2005;62:988–94.

29. Rosenzweig KE, Sura S, Jackson A, et al. Involved-field radiation therapy for inoperable non-small-cell lung cancer. J Clin Oncol 2007;25:5557–61.

30. Vanuytsel LJ, Vansteenkiste JF, Stroobants SG, et al. The impact of (18)F-fluoro-2-deoxy-D-glucose positron emission tomography (FDG-PET) lymph node staging on the radiation treatment volumes in patients with non-small cell lung cancer. Radiother Oncol 2000;55:317–24.

31. Geiger GA, Kim MB, Xanthopoulos EP, et al. Stage migration in planning PET/CT scans in patients due to receive radiotherapy for non-small-cell lung cancer. Clin Lung Cancer 2014;15:79–85.

32. van Baardwijk A, Bosmans G, Boersma L, et al. PET-CT–based auto-contouring in non–small-cell lung cancer correlates with pathology and reduces inter-observer variability in the delineation of the primary tumor and involved nodal volumes. Int J Radiat Oncol Biol Phys 2007;68:771–8.

33. Nestle U, Walter K, Schmidt S, et al. ^{18}F-Deoxyglucose positron emission tomography (FDG-PET) for the planning of radiotherapy in lung cancer: high impact in patients with atelectasis. Int J Radiat Oncol Biol Phys 1999;44:593–7.

34. Houshmand S, Boursi B, Salavati A, et al. Applications of fluorodeoxyglucose PET/computed tomography in the assessment and prediction of radiation therapy-related complications. PET Clin 2015;10:555–71.

35. Chao HH, Berman AT, Simone CB 2nd, et al. Multi-institutional prospective study of reirradiation with proton beam radiotherapy for locoregionally recurrent non-small cell lung cancer. J Thorac Oncol 2017;12:281–92.

36. Verma V, Rwigema JM, Malyapa RS, et al. Systematic assessment of clinical outcomes and toxicities of proton radiotherapy for reirradiation. Radiother Oncol 2017;125:21–30.

37. Wanet M, Delor A, Hanin FX, et al. An individualized radiation dose escalation trial in non-small cell lung cancer based on FDG-PET imaging. Strahlenther Onkol 2017;193:812–22.

38. Kumar SS, Feddock J, Li X, et al. Update of a prospective study of stereotactic body radiation therapy for post-chemoradiation residual disease in Stage II/III non-small cell lung cancer. Int J Radiat Oncol Biol Phys 2017;99:652–9.

39. Veiga C, Janssens G, Teng CL, et al. First clinical investigation of cone beam computed tomography and deformable registration for adaptive proton therapy for lung cancer. Int J Radiat Oncol Biol Phys 2016;95:549–59.

40. Chang JY, Zhang X, Knopf A, et al. Consensus guidelines for implementing pencil-beam scanning proton therapy for thoracic malignancies on behalf of the PTCOG thoracic and lymphoma subcommittee. Int J Radiat Oncol Biol Phys 2017;99:41–50.

41. Kong FM, Ten Haken RK, Schipper M, et al. Effect of midtreatment PET/CT-adapted radiation therapy with concurrent chemotherapy in patients with locally advanced non-small-cell lung cancer: a phase 2 clinical trial. JAMA Oncol 2017;3:1358–65.

42. Ding XP, Zhang J, Li BS, et al. Feasibility of shrinking field radiation therapy through 18F-FDG PET/CT after 40 Gy for stage III non-small cell lung cancers. Asian Pac J Cancer Prev 2012;13:319–23.

43. Ding X, Li H, Wang Z, et al. A clinical study of shrinking field radiation therapy based on (18)FFDG PET/CT for stage III non-small cell lung cancer. Technol Cancer Res Treat 2013;12:251–7.

44. Bradley J, Thorstad WL, Mutic S, et al. Impact of FDG-PET on radiation therapy volume delineation in non-small cell lung cancer. Int J Radiat Oncol Biol Phys 2004;59:78–86.

45. Verma V, Simone CB 2nd, Werner-Wasik M. Acute and late toxicities of concurrent chemoradiotherapy for locally-advanced non-small cell lung cancer. Cancers (Basel) 2017;8:9.

46. Simone CB 2nd. New era in radiation oncology for lung cancer: recognizing the importance of cardiac irradiation. J Clin Oncol 2017;35:1381–3.

47. Haque W, Verma V, Fakhreddine M, et al. Trends in cardiac mortality in patients with locally advanced non-small cell lung cancer. Int J Radiat Oncol Biol Phys 2018;100:470–7.

48. Koh W-J, Abu-Rustum NR, Bean S, et al. Cervical cancer, Version 3.2019, NCCN clinical practice guidelines in oncology. J Natl Compr Cancer Netw 2019;17:64–84.

49. Tsai CS, Chang TC, Lai CH, et al. Preliminary report of using FDG-PET to detect extrapelvic lesions in cervical cancer patients with enlarged pelvic lymph nodes on MRI/CT. Int J Radiat Oncol Biol Phys 2004;58:1506–12.

50. Gee MS, Atri M, Bandos AI, et al. Identification of distant metastatic disease in uterine cervical and endometrial cancers with FDG PET/CT: analysis from the ACRIN 6671/GOG 0233 multicenter trial. Radiology 2018;287:176–84.

51. Esthappan J, Mutic S, Malyapa RS, et al. Treatment planning guidelines regarding the use of CT/PET-guided IMRT for cervical carcinoma with positive paraaortic lymph nodes. Int J Radiat Oncol Biol Phys 2004;58:1289–97.

52. Han K, Croke J, Foltz W, et al. A prospective study of DWI, DCE-MRI and FDG PET imaging for target

delineation in brachytherapy for cervical cancer. Radiother Oncol 2016;120:519–25.

53. Oh D, Huh SJ, Park W, et al. Clinical outcomes in cervical cancer patients treated by FDG-PET/CT-based 3-dimensional planning for the first brachytherapy session. Medicine (Baltimore) 2016;95: e3895.

54. Snyder JE, Willett AB, Sun W, et al. Is SBRT boost feasible for PET positive lymph nodes for cervical cancer? Evaluation using tumor control probability and QUANTEC criteria. Pract Radiat Oncol 2019;9: e156–63.

55. Osborne EM, Klopp AH, Jhingran A, et al. Impact of treatment year on survival and adverse effects in patients with cervical cancer and paraortic lymph node metastases treated with definitive extended-field radiation therapy. Pract Radiat Oncol 2017;7:e165–73.

56. Lin S-Y, Tsai C-S, Chang Y-C, et al. The role of pretreatment FDG-PET in treating cervical cancer patients with enlarged pelvic lymph node(s) shown on MRI: a phase 3 randomized trial with long-term follow-up. Int J Radiat Oncol Biol Phys 2015;92: 577–85.

57. Toya R, Matsuyama T, Saito T, et al. Impact of hybrid FDG-PET/CT on gross tumor volume definition of cervical esophageal cancer: reducing interobserver variation. J Radiat Res 2019;60:348–52.

58. Klopp AH, Moughan J, Portelance L, et al. Hematologic toxicity in RTOG 0418: a phase 2 study of postoperative IMRT for gynecologic cancer. Int J Radiat Oncol Biol Phys 2013;86:83–90.

59. Rose BS, Liang Y, Lau SK, et al. Correlation between radiation dose to (1)(8)F-FDG-PET defined active bone marrow subregions and acute hematologic toxicity in cervical cancer patients treated with chemoradiotherapy. Int J Radiat Oncol Biol Phys 2012; 83:1185–91.

60. Liang Y, Bydder M, Yashar CM, et al. Prospective study of functional bone marrow-sparing intensity modulated radiation therapy with concurrent chemotherapy for pelvic malignancies. Int J Radiat Oncol Biol Phys 2013;85:406–14.

61. Wyss JC, Carmona R, Karunamuni RA, et al. [18 F] Fluoro-2-deoxy-2- d -glucose versus 3′-deoxy-3′-[18 F]fluorothymidine for defining hematopoietically active pelvic bone marrow in gynecologic patients. Radiother Oncol 2016;118:72–8.

62. Zhou YM, Freese C, Meier T, et al. The absolute volume of PET-defined, active bone marrow spared predicts for high grade hematologic toxicity in cervical cancer patients undergoing chemoradiation. Clin Transl Oncol 2018;20:713–8.

63. Li N, Noticewala SS, Williamson CW, et al. Feasibility of atlas-based active bone marrow sparing intensity modulated radiation therapy for cervical cancer. Radiother Oncol 2017;123:325–30.

64. Verma V, Simone CB 2nd, Wahl AO, et al. Proton radiotherapy for gynecologic neoplasms. Acta Oncol 2016;55:1257–65.

65. Jadvar H. Is there a use for FDG-PET in prostate cancer? Semin Nucl Med 2016;46:502–6.

66. Mohler JL, Antonarakis ES, Armstrong AJ, et al. Prostate cancer, Version 2.2019, NCCN clinical practice guidelines in oncology. J Natl Compr Canc Netw 2019;17:479–505.

67. Buchegger F, Garibotto V, Zilli T, et al. First imaging results of an intraindividual comparison of 11C-acetate and 18F-fluorocholine PET/CT in patients with prostate cancer at early biochemical first or second relapse after prostatectomy or radiotherapy. Eur J Nucl Med Mol Imaging 2014;41:68–78.

68. von Eyben FE, Kairemo K. Meta-analysis of (11)C-choline and (18)F-choline PET/CT for management of patients with prostate cancer. Nucl Med Commun 2014;35:221–30.

69. Kitajima K, Murphy RC, Nathan MA, et al. Detection of recurrent prostate cancer after radical prostatectomy: comparison of 11C-Choline PET/CT with pelvic multiparametric MR imaging with endorectal coil. J Nucl Med 2014;55:223–32.

70. Shen C-T, Qiu Z-L, Han T-T, et al. Performance of 18F-Fluoride PET or PET/CT for the detection of bone metastases. Clin Nucl Med 2015;40:103–10.

71. Akin-Akintayo O, Tade F, Mittal P, et al. Prospective evaluation of fluciclovine (18 F) PET-CT and MRI in detection of recurrent prostate cancer in non-prostatectomy patients. Eur J Radiol 2018;102:1–8.

72. Hijazi S, Meller B, Leitsmann C, et al. Pelvic lymph node dissection for nodal oligometastatic prostate cancer detected by [68] Ga-PSMA-positron emission tomography/computerized tomography. Prostate 2015;75:1934–40.

73. Lawhn-Heath C, Flavell RR, Behr SC, et al. Single-center prospective evaluation of [68] Ga-PSMA-11 PET in biochemical recurrence of prostate cancer. Am J Roentgenol 2019. https://doi.org/10.2214/AJR.18.20699.

74. Meredith G, Wong D, Yaxley J, et al. The use of [68] Ga-PSMA PET CT in men with biochemical recurrence after definitive treatment of acinar prostate cancer. BJU Int 2016;118:49–55.

75. McCarthy M, Francis R, Tang C, et al. A multicentre prospective clinical trial of 68Gallium PSMA HBED-CC PET-CT restaging in biochemically relapsed prostate carcinoma: oligometastatic rate and distribution, compared to standard imaging. Int J Radiat Oncol Biol Phys 2019;104:801–8.

76. Boreta L, Gadzinski AJ, Wu SY, et al. Location of recurrence by Gallium-68 PSMA-11 PET scan in prostate cancer patients eligible for salvage radiotherapy. Urology 2019;129:165–71.

77. Fendler WP, Calais J, Eiber M, et al. Assessment of [68] Ga-PSMA-11 PET accuracy in localizing recurrent

prostate cancer. JAMA Oncol 2019. https://doi.org/10.1001/jamaoncol.2019.0096.

78. Calais J, Czernin J, Fendler WP, et al. Randomized prospective phase III trial of 68Ga-PSMA-11 PET/CT molecular imaging for prostate cancer salvage radiotherapy planning [PSMA-SRT]. BMC Cancer 2019;19:18.

79. Schwenck J, Olthof S-C, Pfannenberg C, et al. Intention to treat analysis of [68] Ga-PSMA and [11] C-choline PET/CT versus CT for prostate cancer recurrences after surgery. J Nucl Med 2019. https://doi.org/10.2967/jnumed.118.224543.

80. Jilg CA, Drendel V, Rischke HC, et al. Detection Rate of [18] F-choline-PET/CT and [68] Ga-PSMA-HBED-CC-PET/CT for prostate cancer lymph node metastases with direct link from PET to histopathology: dependence on the size of tumor deposits in lymph nodes. J Nucl Med 2019;60:971–7.

81. Walacides D, Meier A, Knöchelmann AC, et al. Comparison of 68 Ga-PSMA ligand PET/CT versus conventional cross-sectional imaging for target volume delineation for metastasis-directed radiotherapy for metachronous lymph node metastases from prostate cancer. Strahlenther Onkol 2019;195:420–9.

82. Jani AB, Schreibmann E, Rossi PJ, et al. Impact of [18] F-Fluciclovine PET on target volume definition for postprostatectomy salvage radiotherapy: initial findings from a randomized trial. J Nucl Med 2017;58:412–8.

83. Schreibmann E, Schuster DM, Rossi PJ, et al. Image guided planning for prostate carcinomas with incorporation of anti-3-[18F]FACBC (Fluciclovine) positron emission tomography: workflow and initial findings from a randomized trial. Int J Radiat Oncol Biol Phys 2016;96:206–13.

84. Cheson BD, Fisher RI, Barrington SF, et al. Recommendations for initial evaluation, staging, and response assessment of Hodgkin and non-Hodgkin lymphoma: the Lugano classification. J Clin Oncol 2014;32:3059–68.

85. Hoppe RT, Advani RH, Ai WZ, et al. NCCN guidelines insights: hodgkin lymphoma, version 1.2018. J Natl Compr Canc Netw 2018;16:245–54.

86. Illidge T, Specht L, Yahalom J, et al. Modern radiation therapy for nodal non-Hodgkin lymphoma-target definition and dose guidelines from the International Lymphoma Radiation Oncology Group. Int J Radiat Oncol Biol Phys 2014;89:49–58.

87. Specht L, Yahalom J, Illidge T, et al. Modern radiation therapy for Hodgkin lymphoma: field and dose guidelines from the international lymphoma radiation oncology group (ILROG). Int J Radiat Oncol Biol Phys 2014;89:854–62.

88. Yahalom J, Illidge T, Specht L, et al. Modern radiation therapy for extranodal lymphomas: field and dose guidelines from the international lymphoma radiation oncology group. Int J Radiat Oncol Biol Phys 2015;92:11–31.

89. André MPE, Girinsky T, Federico M, et al. Early positron emission tomography response–adapted treatment in stage I and II hodgkin lymphoma: final results of the randomized EORTC/LYSA/FIL H10 trial. J Clin Oncol 2017;35:1786–94.

90. Radford J, Illidge T, Counsell N, et al. Results of a trial of PET-directed therapy for early-stage Hodgkin's lymphoma. N Engl J Med 2015;372:1598–607.

91. Pfreundschuh M, Christofyllakis K, Altmann B, et al. Radiotherapy to bulky disease pet-negative after immunochemotherapy can be spared in elderly dlbcl patients: results of a planned interim analysis of the first 187 patients with bulky disease treated in the optimal >60 study of the dshnhl. Hematol Oncol 2017;35:129–30.

92. Ferdova E, Ferda J, Baxa J. 18F-FDG-PET/MRI in lymphoma patients. Eur J Radiol 2017;94:A52–63.

93. Mena E, Lindenberg ML, Turkbey BI, et al. A pilot study of the value of 18F-fluoro-deoxy-thymidine PET/CT in predicting viable lymphoma in residual 18F-FDG avid masses after completion of therapy. Clin Nucl Med 2014;39:874–81.

94. Zanoni L, Broccoli A, Lambertini A, et al. Role of 18F-FLT PET/CT in suspected recurrent or residual lymphoma: final results of a pilot prospective trial. Eur J Nucl Med Mol Imaging 2019;46:1661–71.

95. Luo Y, Cao X, Pan Q, et al. ^{68}Ga-pentixafor PET/CT for imaging of chemokine receptor-4 expression in Waldenström macroglobulinemia/lymphoplasmacytic lymphoma: comparison to [18] F-FDG PET/CT. J Nucl Med 2019. https://doi.org/10.2967/jnumed.119.226134.

96. Kaste SC, Snyder SE, Metzger ML, et al. Comparison of [11] C-methionine and [18] F-FDG PET/CT for staging and follow-up of pediatric lymphoma. J Nucl Med 2017;58:419–24.

97. Muylle K, Flamen P, Vugts DJ, et al. Tumour targeting and radiation dose of radioimmunotherapy with (90) Y-rituximab in CD20+ B-cell lymphoma as predicted by (89)Zr-rituximab immuno-PET: impact of preloading with unlabelled rituximab. Eur J Nucl Med Mol Imaging 2015;42:1304–14.

18F-Fluorodeoxyglucose PET in Locally Advanced Non–small Cell Lung Cancer
From Predicting Outcomes to Guiding Therapy

N. Patrik Brodin, PhD[a,b,*], Wolfgang A. Tomé, PhD[a,b,c],
Tony Abraham, DO, MPA[d], Nitin Ohri, MD[a,b]

KEYWORDS

• PET • Non–small cell lung cancer • Radiation therapy

KEY POINTS

- PET using 18-fluorodeoxyglucose (FDG) has been established as an important part of the prognosis, radiation therapy target definition, and treatment evaluation for locally advanced non–small cell lung cancer (NSCLC), and new avenues continue to be discovered for how to use this technology to best treat these patients.
- FDG-PET has taken on several key roles in the treatment of locally advanced NSCLC, and additional uses for PET are being studied.
- Pretreatment metabolic tumor volume and total lesion glycolysis are independent predictors of treatment outcome, in some reports more so than disease stage.
- There is some complementary information to be gained from pretreatment compared with interim FDG-PET scans and studying these dynamics could lead to more individualized treatment options.

INTRODUCTION

Despite recent technological and biological advances in its treatment, lung cancer remains the leading cause of cancer-related death. Broadly, most lung cancers are classified as non–small cell lung cancer (NSCLC).[1] Locally advanced disease (a term that typically includes stage III disease, unresectable stage II disease, and possibly oligometastatic disease in which the metastases have been treated aggressively) comprises approximately 20% to 30% of all NSCLC cases.[2]

One of the paramount technical advances for NSCLC in the last 4 decades is the advent of 18-fluorodeoxyglucose (FDG) PET. Initially, the utility of FDG-PET was mainly to aid in identification and classification of suspicious lymph node regions, and now PET combined with computed tomography (CT) as integrated PET/CT has become a mainstay component in the staging and work-up of patients with NSCLC receiving chemoradiotherapy (CRT).[3–9]

More recently, there has been a great interest in trying to determine the prognostic value of

[a] Institute for Onco-Physics, Albert Einstein College of Medicine, Bronx, NY 10461, USA; [b] Department of Radiation Oncology, Montefiore Medical Center, Bronx, NY 10461, USA; [c] Department of Neurology, Albert Einstein College of Medicine, Bronx, NY 10461, USA; [d] Department of Radiology (Nuclear Medicine), Albert Einstein College of Medicine, Bronx, NY 10461, USA
* Corresponding author. Institute for Onco-Physics, Albert Einstein College of Medicine, Montefiore Medical Center, 1300 Morris Park Avenue, Block Building Room 104, Bronx, NY 10461, USA.
E-mail address: patrik.brodin@einstein.yu.edu

PET Clin 15 (2020) 55–63
https://doi.org/10.1016/j.cpet.2019.08.009
1556-8598/20/© 2019 Elsevier Inc. All rights reserved.

features related to the FDG-PET uptake of primary NSCLC tumors. This interest includes using metrics such as standardized uptake value (SUV) for measuring tumor response,[10–12] and deriving image features based on the spatial distribution of the FDG-PET uptake throughout the tumor.[13–16] The role of FDG-PET in locally advanced NSCLC is evolving, and more quantitative analytical approaches are being extensively pursued. The value of posttreatment or intermediate PET scans to further individualize therapy is also being investigated in a variety of approaches.[17,18] This article provides a review of the clinical evidence detailing the use of FDG-PET for target volume definition, prognostication of survival and tumor control, and guiding radiation therapy (RT) through risk adaptation and dose escalation for patients with NSCLC treated with definitive RT, including RT combined with sequential or concurrent chemotherapy.

THE PROGNOSTIC VALUE OF ^{18}F-FLUORODEOXYGLUCOSE PET
Pretreatment Volumetric and standardized uptake value–based Predictors of Prognosis

A variety of metrics can be extracted from the pretreatment FDG-PET images, with the most common being SUV-based markers or markers related to metabolic tumor volume (MTV). For SUV, these values are calculated per voxel as the ratio of the activity concentration in a voxel compared with the whole-body concentration of the administered activity. In contrast, MTV is defined as the volume of voxels within a metabolically active lesion, either contoured by hand or semiautomatically contoured based on certain SUV thresholding algorithms. Frequently reported metrics include SUV_{mean}, SUV_{max}, SUV_{peak}, MTV, and total lesion glycolysis (TLG; defined as SUV_{mean} multiplied by MTV, sometimes referred to as total glycolytic activity). For early-stage disease, strong correlations would generally be expected between volumetric markers such as MTV and SUV-based markers, simply because smaller tumors often do not display very high SUV values. For locally advanced disease, there is a better chance of teasing out the independent prognostic effect of these different markers because of reduced volume dependence.

To that end, several studies have shown a survival benefit for patients with lower pretreatment SUV_{max},[19–24] with suggested cutoff values ranging from 5.4 to 15.

Note that, out of these studies, 2 showed a significant association between SUV_{max} and tumor size,[20,22] whereas several others did not assess

this association or the prognostic value of volume-based parameters such as MTV and TLG.[19,21,23] This omission makes it difficult to appreciably determine the independent prognostic value of pretreatment SUV-based metrics for locally advanced NSCLC, because tumor volume is a strong confounder for the association with survival in this disease. This point is exemplified by a study from the MAASTRO group in which pretreatment SUV_{max} remained a significant prognostic factor in multivariable analysis, but tumor volume was clearly the dominant factor on univariable analyses.[24]

As far as volume-based parameters are concerned, there have also been many studies showing a significant association between pretreatment MTV or TLG and survival,[25–30] as well as local disease progression.[28,31,32] There is naturally a strong correlation between MTV and TLG, and different investigators have chosen to report on either one of these or both, but including both in the same multivariable analysis is not recommended because of issues with colinearity. For local disease progression, pretreatment MTV was a univariable prognostic factor in 1 study (hazard ratio [HR] = 1.53; P = .049),[31] and another study examining an MTV cutoff value showed 45% 2-year local progression if MTV was greater than 25 cm^3 versus 5% if MTV was less than 25 cm^3.[28] This finding was later validated in an independent cohort confirming the prognostic value of a 25 cm^3 MTV cutoff (HR = 6.6; P = .008).[32] Importantly, SUV_{max} was also examined as a prognostic factor in these studies and was found to have little association with risk of death (HR = 1.02; P = .41)[31] and was outperformed by MTV as a predictor of local disease progression (area under the curve for MTV [AUC_{MTV}] = 0.827 vs AUC_{SUVmax} = 0.763).[28]

American college of radiology imaging network (ACRIN) 6668/Radiation Therapy Oncology Group (RTOG) 0235 was a large, multi-institutional study in which patients with stage II to III NSCLC underwent PET before and 12 to 16 weeks after finishing CRT. The primary objective was to show the prognostic value of posttreatment PET activity (peak SUV). In a secondary analysis of this trial, pretreatment MTV was shown to be an independent predictor of overall survival (OS) (HR = 1.04 per 10 cm^3 increase; P<.001), whereas SUV_{max} was not (HR = 1.00; P = .64).[27] Another study of 28 patients found a significant worsening in progression-free survival (PFS) with increasing pretreatment TLG (HR = 1.047 per 10-unit increase; P = .009), with a baseline TLG greater than or equal to 450 indicating worse prognosis.[29] These investigators did not find any significant association between PFS and pretreatment SUV_{mean} ($P = .575$) or SUV_{max} ($P = .447$). A similar study also found no significant association between SUV_{max} and PFS, but it did reveal a significant difference in median PFS of 14.3 months with pretreatment MTV less than 60 cm^3 compared with 9.7 months for MTV greater than 60 cm^3 ($P = .03$).[28] In a meta-analysis of 13 studies of patients with NSCLC (all using different cutoff values for pretreatment FDG-PET metrics), a strong association was found with OS for both MTV (pooled HR = 2.31; $P<.001$) and TLG (pooled HR = 2.43; $P<.001$) as well as a slightly weaker association with SUV_{max} (HR = 1.20; $P = .008$).[26]

Several of the studies of pretreatment prognostic PET metrics either accounted for tumor stage in their analysis[19,22,26] or found an association with treatment outcomes in which stage was not a significant predictor.[24,30] This finding suggests that pretreatment PET metrics provide potential for treatment stratification and prognostication beyond classic tumor staging.

Interim and Posttreatment PET-based Predictors of Prognosis

There has been a lot of interest in studying the prognostic value of changes in PET metrics from pretreatment to midtreatment or posttreatment to identify signals to guide adaptive treatment. One of the first studies to show the utility of midtreatment PET came from the Michigan group in 2007 and showed that the metabolic tumor response during treatment, based on peak FDG activity, was a promising early response marker, because it was strongly correlated with values seen on scans 3 to 4 months after treatment ($R^2 = 0.7$; $P<.001$).[33] In a series of patients who underwent CRT followed by resection for superior sulcus tumors, change in SUV_{max} from before to after treatment was a powerful predictor of pathologic complete response or major response (<10% viable tumor cells after CRT).[34] Similarly, higher posttreatment SUV_{max} (or SUV_{peak}, because these were found to be interchangeable) was associated with worse OS after concurrent CRT (multivariable HR = 1.087; $P<.001$), with an optimal SUV_{max} cutoff value of 5.0 ($P = .02$).[35] This finding can be compared with the study by French investigators that found an optimal cutoff for SUV_{max} after 5 weeks of treatment of 5.3 for predicting disease-free survival at 1 year.[36] In contrast, 1 study did not find a significant association between changes in any PET metrics from pretreatment to midtreatment and OS in an analysis of 28 patients with stage III to IV NSCLC.[37] One study examined the change in SUV_{mean} from

pretreatment to the second week of treatment and found that the 2-year OS was 92% if the ΔSUV_{mean} was greater than or equal to 15% versus only 33% if the ΔSUV_{mean} was less than 15% ($P = .004$), whereas pretreatment PET metrics alone did not hold prognostic value for OS.[38]

A few studies found the change in MTV from pretreatment to posttreatment or midtreatment to have prognostic value, with 1 showing a median OS of 36.5 months if $\Delta MTV_{pre/mid}$ was greater than 29.7% versus 18.0 months if $\Delta MTV_{pre/mid}$ was less than 29.7% in 53 patients with NSCLC treated with concurrent CRT.[39] A similar result was found in a German study of 65 patients that reported a median PFS of 14 months if $\Delta MTV_{mid/post}$ was greater than 15% versus 7 months if $\Delta MTV_{mid/post}$ was less than 15%.[40] Another study stratified patients according to risk groups based on changes in TLG from pretreatment to the second week of treatment, with baseline TLG less than 500 and ΔTLG greater than or equal to 38% constituting those with favorable PFS and TLG greater than or equal to 450 and ΔTLG less than 38% as the unfavorable risk category.[29]

^{18}F-Fluorodeoxyglucose PET Textural Image Features for Predicting Treatment Outcomes

Using textural image features derived from FDG-PET scans has been an area of intense research in the last few years, with several studies focusing on NSCLC. Before discussing these studies, it is prudent to recognize some important pitfalls when studying image features as biomarkers. A large number of features can be derived from a single PET scan of a lung tumor, and statistical problems with multiple testing and high false-discovery rates can be an issue if not appropriately accounted for, akin to multiple testing concerns of PET SUV parameters when predicting survival.[41] This pitfall was highlighted in a recent review article showing an average 76% type-I error probability among 15 studies on PET and CT textural image features as predictors of outcome.[42] Furthermore, the stability and reproducibility of textural image features can be an issue when used as prognostic markers, which was recently tested by the MAASTRO group.[43] Eleven patients were used for a test-retest comparison and 23 patients for an investigation of interobserver variability, with most of the tested features showing high test-retest (71%) and interobserver (91%) stability, based on intraclass correlation coefficient.

Another important point to address is the correlation that is often found between image features representing tumor heterogeneity and MTV, because larger tumors typically show higher levels of heterogeneity. A French study investigated whether MTV and features of tumor heterogeneity provided complementary prognostic information, or simply described the same part of the variance in patient outcome.[14] Heterogeneity and MTV were both independent prognostic factors for OS (P = .009 and P = .005, respectively), but more so for larger tumors. For small tumors, there was considerable correlation between MTV and heterogeneity, and the investigators suggest that there may be complementary prognostic information for tumors greater than 10 cm^3, and increasingly so with increasing tumor size. This finding was corroborated by a secondary analysis of ACRIN 6668/RTOG 0235 that found the SumMean textural feature to be an independent predictor of OS.[15] Tumors with SumMean less than or equal to 0.018 were considered more heterogeneous and were associated with worse OS, but only for large tumors with MTV greater than 93.3 cm^3 (P<.001).

In a study from Kings College, high NSCLC tumor coarseness was associated with worse OS and PFS (P = .003 and P = .002), whereas PFS durations were longer in patients whose tumors showed high levels of contrast and busyness (P = .015 and P = .02).[44] A Swedish study developed a novel marker based on longitudinal pattern features derived from voxel-wise changes from pretreatment to midtreatment PET scans, with AUCs for predicting 2-year OS of 0.96 and 0.93 for patients with NSCLC receiving sequential and concurrent CRT, respectively.[45] One study evaluated the change in textural PET features comparing pretreatment features with those following 40 Gy of concurrent CRT.[46] Change in textural features performed better than baseline features with higher sensitivity (92% vs 73%) and specificity (84% vs 80%), and change in the contrast feature was an independent predictor of PFS (multivariable HR = 0.48; P = .021) and OS (multivariable HR = 0.52; P = .015). As with locally advanced NSCLC, radiomic features were shown to correlate with OS (P = .003) and freedom from nodal failure (P = .038) in an analysis of 100 patients treated with stereotactic body RT for early-stage NSCLC.[47]

^{18}F-FLUORODEOXYGLUCOSE PET TO GUIDE RADIATION THERAPY
The Addition of PET to Radiation Therapy Target Delineation

The use of combined PET/CT is now commonplace in most centers that treat NSCLC with RT,

and the addition of PET has been shown to considerably alter the RT gross tumor volume (GTV) target, both for the primary tumor and involved lymph nodes.[48–52] In a study of 21 patients with NSCLC, investigators showed that the information obtained for target volume delineation from PET is complementary to that from CT alone, with larger CT-GTVs in 48% of cases and larger PET-GTVs in 33% of cases.[53] Another study found that marginal misses would have occurred in 3 of 10 NSCLC cases had PET not been used to define the target volume.[54] That study also found a reduction in lung V20 (percentage of the lungs receiving 20 Gy) in 4 patients when PET was used, again showing that the use of PET can result in smaller target volumes, which have a potential to reduce treatment-related toxicities. A small study of 5 patients with NSCLC showed that using CT alone would have underdosed the PET-based planning target volume (PTV) in 2 patients, with minimum PTV doses ranging from 12% to 63% of the prescribed dose.[55]

RTOG 0515 compared target delineation for stage II or III NSCLC with and without PET and found that including the PET information resulted in smaller GTVs compared with using CT alone (86.2 vs 98.7 cm^3; P<.001).[50] PET-based target volume definition does not lead to consistently smaller or larger GTVs compared with using CT when examining different studies, but leads to a change in target volume that is different between individual patients. In a study of 14 patients with NSCLC, the addition of PET led to a smaller GTV definition in 12 of 14 patients compared with using CT alone.[56] In contrast, a study from investigators from Wisconsin in 2009 showed that including PET imaging for target delineation resulted in a larger GTV in 17 (47%) patients with lung cancer, compared with a smaller GTV in 19 (53%) patients, with 11 of 36 patients having a major change to the RT plan based on the addition of PET.[57] An analysis of 28 patients with lung cancer receiving either induction chemotherapy followed by RT (n = 14) or RT alone (n = 14) showed that the interobserver variability in GTV definition among 4 oncologists was significantly lower with PET/CT compared with CT alone (P = .032).[58] The addition of PET also led to, on average, larger GTVs for the patients receiving RT alone (19% increase), compared with an average 5% decrease in GTVs for patients receiving induction chemotherapy and RT.

A known issue with RT target volume definition using PET is the variability inherent to the uptake of functional imaging tracers and the dependence on scanner type and background level. To this end, thresholding algorithms are often used to reduce the variability in tumor delineation. A phantom study using spheres of different diameters showed that higher threshold levels were required to accurately render smaller spheres, and this relationship was most clearly shown for low levels of background pixel intensity.[59] Similarly, a French group using an image set of 65 lung cancer lesions from 54 patients showed that that an adaptive thresholding technique was able to accurately measure the size of those lesions with a diameter greater than or equal to 20 mm.[60] For lesions greater than or equal to 20 mm, the average percentage difference and standard deviation between the PET-derived diameter and that derived from histologic examination was 0.8% ($\pm$9.0%), compared with an average 24.7% ($\pm$22.1%) overestimation using PET for lesions less than 20 mm.

PET to Guide Radiation Therapy Dose Escalation

In the last few years there have been several investigations into the potential of using PET to guide nonuniform dose escalation (also referred to as dose painting) strategies, with the aim of improving local tumor control and survival without causing excessive treatment-related toxicities. Dose escalation based on pretreatment PET scans has been explored in a few studies, including a treatment planning study from 2011 showing that it would be feasible to escalate the dose to the PET-positive GTV to 79.2 Gy using a simultaneous integrated boost strategy, with only a small increase in mean lung dose and lung V20.[61] Taking this concept into clinical reality, in a small prospective study of 13 patients with stage II to III NSCLC, 62.5 Gy in 25 fractions was delivered to the CT-based PTV, while boosting the PET-PTV until predefined organ-at-risk constraints were reached.[62] With an average dose to the PET-PTV of 82.1 Gy ($\pm$17.9 Gy), the 1-year and 2-year local PFS rates were 76.9% and 52.8%, respectively, although 2 grade 5 toxicities were observed. PET-based dose painting was further explored in another study using a systematic approach in which an MTV of 25 cm³ was used as a cutoff for high-risk lesions, prescribed to 65 Gy in 25 fractions, whereas smaller lesions received 57 Gy or 52.5 Gy, all in combination with concurrent chemotherapy.[63] The 2-year cumulative incidence of local progression was 15%, with a 2-year OS of 52% and no observed grade 5 toxicities.

Table 1
Summary of studies that implement PET-based dose escalation strategies

Reference	Patients	Dose Escalation	Treatment Outcome	Toxicity
Wanet et al,[62] 2017	13 pt with stage II–III NSCLC treated with concurrent or sequential CRT	62.5 Gy in 25 fx to CT-based PTV with average 82.1 Gy to PET-PTV (max 4.8 Gy/fx)	2-y LPFS was 52.8% with 2 out of 13 local failures. After median 29-mo FU, 54% of patients were still alive	3 cases of grade 3 esophagitis and 2 patients with central tumors had late grade 5 toxicity and died of hemoptysis
Ohri et al,[63] 2018	35 pt with stage IIB–III NSCLC treated with concurrent CRT	65 Gy in 25 fx to lesions with MTV >25 cm³, 57 Gy or 52.5 Gy to lesions with MTV <25 cm³	2-y PFS and OS were 23% and 52%, respectively; 2-y local progression incidence was 15%	No grade 5 toxicity and grade 4 events were hematologic. Nonhematologic grade 3 toxicity observed in 43% of patients
Kong et al,[64] 2017	42 pt with stage II–III NSCLC, 39 of which treated with concurrent CRT	Residual disease on midtreatment PET up to 86 Gy in 30 fx while keeping MLD <20 Gy, with pre-RT PTV and CTV receiving at least 50 Gy and 60 Gy	2-y PFS and OS were 31% and 52%, respectively. Local failure was observed in 6 patients (14%)	12% grade 3 pneumonitis and 7% grade 3 esophagitis, whereas 4 patients died of hemorrhaging, 2 clearly from the lung

Abbreviations: CTV, clinical target volume; FU, follow-up; fx, fractions; LPFS, local PFS; max, maximum; MLD, mean lung dose; pt, patients..

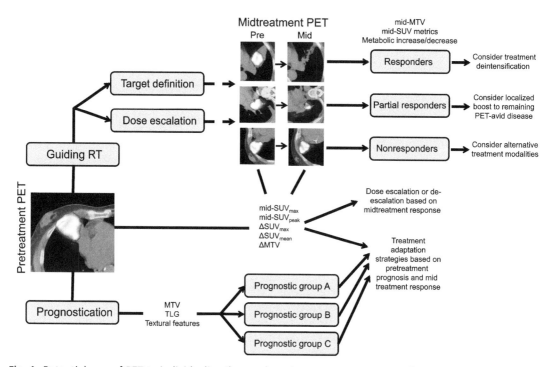

Fig. 1. Potential uses of PET to individualize therapy based on pretreatment as well as interim PET scans.

Treatment adaptation based on midtreatment PET response is another promising strategy that has recently been explored. In a phase II trial of 42 patients with stage II to III NSCLC, dose escalation of residual disease on midtreatment PET up to 86 Gy in 30 fractions was performed, keeping the mean lung dose less than 20 Gy.[64] The 2-year locoregional control rate was 62% and the 2-year OS was 52%, with only 6 out of 42 patients experiencing local failure. **Table 1** summarizes the prospective studies implementing PET-based dose escalation covered in this article.

In an attempt to further stratify patients for dose escalation based on FDG-PET image features, a group from MD Anderson retrospectively analyzed subgroups of patients with NSCLC treated with 60, 70, or 74 Gy.[65] For tumors with high levels of disease solidity and primary co-occurrence matrix energy, patients receiving 74 Gy had better OS ($P = .011$) and PFS ($P = .021$), whereas, for tumors with low levels of these image features, patients receiving 60 to 70 Gy had better OS ($P = .020$) and PFS ($P = .025$) compared with those receiving 74 Gy.

SUMMARY

FDG-PET has taken on several key roles in the treatment of locally advanced NSCLC, and additional uses for PET are being studied. This article summarizes some of the latest advances showing that pretreatment MTV or TLG are independent predictors of treatment outcome, in some reports more so than disease stage. There is clearly some complementary information to be gained from pretreatment compared with interim FDG-PET scans, which may be especially important for smaller tumors, in which the pretreatment PET metrics such as SUV_{max} may be strongly correlated with tumor volume, whereas the interim or posttreatment metrics may indicate response to treatment. Furthermore, it seems that features representing heterogeneity in the tumor PET uptake are important factors to consider for potential treatment stratification, because they have been shown to carry complimentary information to MTV or TLG.

At present, one of the main clinical implementations of FDG-PET for NSCLC consists of aiding target delineation by complementing the RT planning CT scan. **Fig. 1** shows the avenues covered in this article for how PET could be used to individualize and tailor NSCLC treatment. In summary, FDG-PET has been established as an important part of the prognosis, RT target definition, and dynamic treatment adaptation for locally advanced NSCLC, and new avenues continue to be discovered for how to use this technology to best treat these patients.

REFERENCES

1. Siegel RL, Miller KD, Jemal A. Cancer statistics, 2019. CA Cancer J Clin 2019;69:7–34.

2. Tabchi S, Kassouf E, Rassy EE, et al. Management of stage III non-small cell lung cancer. Semin Oncol 2017;44:163–77.

3. De Ruysscher D, Belderbos J, Reymen B, et al. State of the art radiation therapy for lung cancer 2012: a glimpse of the future. Clin Lung Cancer 2013;14:89–95.

4. Gregoire V, Haustermans K, Geets X, et al. PET-based treatment planning in radiotherapy: a new standard? J Nucl Med 2007;48(Suppl 1):68s–77s.

5. Grootjans W, de Geus-Oei LF, Bussink J. Image-guided adaptive radiotherapy in patients with locally advanced non-small cell lung cancer: the art of PET. Q J Nucl Med Mol Imaging 2018;62:369–84.

6. Mac Manus MP. Use of PET/CT for staging and radiation therapy planning in patients with non-small cell lung cancer. Q J Nucl Med Mol Imaging 2010;54:510–20.

7. Usmanij EA, de Geus-Oei LF, Bussink J, et al. Update on F-18-fluoro-deoxy-glucose-PET/computed tomography in nonsmall cell lung cancer. Curr Opin Pulm Med 2015;21:314–21.

8. van Loon J, van Baardwijk A, Boersma L, et al. Therapeutic implications of molecular imaging with PET in the combined modality treatment of lung cancer. Cancer Treat Rev 2011;37:331–43.

9. Geiger GA, Kim MB, Xanthopoulos EP, et al. Stage migration in planning PET/CT scans in patients due to receive radiotherapy for non-small-cell lung cancer. Clin Lung Cancer 2014;15(1):79–85.

10. Allen-Auerbach M, Weber WA. Measuring response with FDG-PET: methodological aspects. Oncologist 2009;14:369–77.

11. Hicks RJ. Role of 18F-FDG PET in assessment of response in non-small cell lung cancer. J Nucl Med 2009;50(Suppl 1):31s–42s.

12. Rosenzweig KE, Fox JL, Giraud P. Response to radiation. Semin Radiat Oncol 2004;14:322–5.

13. Aerts HJ, Velazquez ER, Leijenaar RT, et al. Decoding tumour phenotype by noninvasive imaging using a quantitative radiomics approach. Nat Commun 2014;5:4006.

14. Hatt M, Majdoub M, Vallieres M, et al. 18F-FDG PET uptake characterization through texture analysis: investigating the complementary nature of heterogeneity and functional tumor volume in a multi-cancer site patient cohort. J Nucl Med 2015;56:38–44.

15. Ohri N, Duan F, Snyder BS, et al. Pretreatment 18F-FDG PET textural features in locally advanced non-small cell lung cancer: secondary analysis of ACRIN 6668/RTOG 0235. J Nucl Med 2016;57:842–8.

16. Sollini M, Cozzi L, Antunovic L, et al. PET Radiomics in NSCLC: state of the art and a proposal for harmonization of methodology. Sci Rep 2017;7:358.

17. Cremonesi M, Gilardi L, Ferrari ME, et al. Role of interim (18)F-FDG-PET/CT for the early prediction of clinical outcomes of Non-Small Cell Lung Cancer (NSCLC) during radiotherapy or chemo-radiotherapy. A systematic review. Eur J Nucl Med Mol Imaging 2017;44:1915–27.

18. Kased N, Erasmus JJ, Komaki R, et al. Prognostic value of posttreatment [18F] fluorodeoxyglucose uptake of primary non-small cell lung carcinoma treated with radiation therapy with or without chemotherapy: a brief review. J Thorac Oncol 2008;3:534–8.

19. Borst GR, Belderbos JS, Boellaard R, et al. Standardised FDG uptake: a prognostic factor for inoperable non-small cell lung cancer. Eur J Cancer 2005;41:1533–41.

20. Masarykova A, Scepanovic D, Povinec P, et al. Tumour metabolic activity measured by fluorodeoxyglucose positron emission tomography for radiotherapy planning as a prognostic factor for locally advanced non-small cell lung cancer. Bratisl Lek Listy 2018;119:133–8.

21. Ohno Y, Koyama H, Yoshikawa T, et al. Diffusion-weighted MRI versus 18F-FDG PET/CT: performance as predictors of tumor treatment response and patient survival in patients with non-small cell lung cancer receiving chemoradiotherapy. AJR Am J Roentgenol 2012;198:75–82.

22. Tong AN, Han SR, Yan P, et al. Prognostic value of FDG uptake in primary inoperable non-small cell lung cancer. Med Oncol 2014;31:780.

23. Ulger S, Demirci NY, Eroglu FN, et al. High FDG uptake predicts poorer survival in locally advanced nonsmall cell lung cancer patients undergoing curative radiotherapy, independently of tumor size. J Cancer Res Clin Oncol 2014;140:495–502.

24. Velazquez ER, Aerts HJ, Oberije C, et al. Prediction of residual metabolic activity after treatment in NSCLC patients. Acta Oncol 2010;49:1033–9.

25. Salavati A, Duan F, Snyder BS, et al. Optimal FDG PET/CT volumetric parameters for risk stratification in patients with locally advanced non-small cell lung cancer: results from the ACRIN 6668/RTOG 0235 trial. Eur J Nucl Med Mol Imaging 2017;44(12):1969–83.

26. Im HJ, Pak K, Cheon GJ, et al. Prognostic value of volumetric parameters of (18)F-FDG PET in non-small-cell lung cancer: a meta-analysis. Eur J Nucl Med Mol Imaging 2015;42:241–51.

27. Ohri N, Duan F, Machtay M, et al. Pretreatment FDG-PET metrics in stage III non-small cell lung cancer: ACRIN 6668/RTOG 0235. J Natl Cancer Inst 2015; 107 [pii:djv004].

28. Ohri N, Piperdi B, Garg MK, et al. Pre-treatment FDG-PET predicts the site of in-field progression following concurrent chemoradiotherapy for stage III non-small cell lung cancer. Lung Cancer 2015; 87:23–7.

29. Usmanij EA, de Geus-Oei LF, Troost EG, et al. 18F-FDG PET early response evaluation of locally advanced non-small cell lung cancer treated with concomitant chemoradiotherapy. J Nucl Med 2013; 54:1528–34.

30. Wang D, Koh ES, Descallar J, et al. Application of novel quantitative techniques for fluorodeoxyglucose positron emission tomography/computed tomography in patients with non-small-cell lung cancer. Asia Pac J Clin Oncol 2016;12:349–58.

31. Gensheimer MF, Hong JC, Chang-Halpenny C, et al. Mid-radiotherapy PET/CT for prognostication and detection of early progression in patients with stage III non-small cell lung cancer. Radiother Oncol 2017; 125:338–43.

32. Ohri N, Bodner WR, Halmos B, et al. (18)F-Fluorodeoxyglucose/Positron emission tomography predicts patterns of failure after definitive chemoradiation therapy for locally advanced non-small cell lung cancer. Int J Radiat Oncol Biol Phys 2017;97: 372–80.

33. Kong FM, Frey KA, Quint LE, et al. A pilot study of [18F]fluorodeoxyglucose positron emission tomography scans during and after radiation-based therapy in patients with non small-cell lung cancer. J Clin Oncol 2007;25:3116–23.

34. Bahce I, Vos CG, Dickhoff C, et al. Metabolic activity measured by FDG PET predicts pathological response in locally advanced superior sulcus NSCLC. Lung Cancer 2014;85:205–12.

35. Machtay M, Duan F, Siegel BA, et al. Prediction of survival by [18F]fluorodeoxyglucose positron emission tomography in patients with locally advanced non-small-cell lung cancer undergoing definitive chemoradiation therapy: results of the ACRIN 6668/RTOG 0235 trial. J Clin Oncol 2013;31: 3823–30.

36. Vera P, Mezzani-Saillard S, Edet-Sanson A, et al. FDG PET during radiochemotherapy is predictive of outcome at 1 year in non-small-cell lung cancer patients: a prospective multicentre study (RTEP2). Eur J Nucl Med Mol Imaging 2014;41:1057–65.

37. Lazzeroni M, Uhrdin J, Carvalho S, et al. Evaluation of third treatment week as temporal window for assessing responsiveness on repeated FDG-PET-CT scans in Non-Small Cell Lung Cancer patients. Phys Med 2018;46:45–51.

38. van Elmpt W, Ollers M, Dingemans AM, et al. Response assessment using 18F-FDG PET early in the course of radiotherapy correlates with survival in advanced-stage non-small cell lung cancer. J Nucl Med 2012;53:1514–20.

39. Huang W, Fan M, Liu B, et al. Value of metabolic tumor volume on repeated 18F-FDG PET/CT for early prediction of survival in locally advanced non-small cell lung cancer treated with concurrent chemoradiotherapy. J Nucl Med 2014;55:1584–90.

40. Roengvoraphoj O, Wijaya C, Eze C, et al. Analysis of primary tumor metabolic volume during chemoradiotherapy in locally advanced non-small cell lung cancer. Strahlenther Onkol 2018;194:107–15.

41. Berman AT, Ellenberg SS, Simone CB 2nd. Predicting survival in non-small-cell lung cancer using positron emission tomography: several conclusions from multiple comparisons. J Clin Oncol 2014;32(15): 1631–2.

42. Chalkidou A, O'Doherty MJ, Marsden PK. False discovery rates in PET and CT studies with texture features: a systematic review. PLoS One 2015;10: e0124165.

43. Leijenaar RT, Carvalho S, Velazquez ER, et al. Stability of FDG-PET Radiomics features: an integrated analysis of test-retest and inter-observer variability. Acta Oncol 2013;52:1391–7.

44. Cook GJ, Yip C, Siddique M, et al. Are pretreatment 18F-FDG PET tumor textural features in non-small cell lung cancer associated with response and survival after chemoradiotherapy? J Nucl Med 2013; 54:19–26.

45. Buizza G, Toma-Dasu I, Lazzeroni M, et al. Early tumor response prediction for lung cancer patients using novel longitudinal pattern features from sequential PET/CT image scans. Phys Med 2018; 54:21–9.

46. Dong X, Sun X, Sun L, et al. Early change in metabolic tumor heterogeneity during chemoradiotherapy and its prognostic value for patients with locally advanced non-small cell lung cancer. PLoS One 2016;11:e0157836.

47. Li H, Galperin-Aizenberg M, Pryma D, et al. Unsupervised machine learning of radiomic features for predicting treatment response and overall survival of early stage non-small cell lung cancer patients treated with stereotactic body radiation therapy. Radiother Oncol 2018;129(2):218–26.

48. Verma V, Choi JI, Sawant A, et al. Use of PET and other functional imaging to guide target delineation in radiation oncology. Semin Radiat Oncol 2018; 28(3):171–7.

49. Ashamalla H, Rafla S, Parikh K, et al. The contribution of integrated PET/CT to the evolving definition of treatment volumes in radiation treatment planning in lung cancer. Int J Radiat Oncol Biol Phys 2005;63: 1016–23.

50. Bradley J, Bae K, Choi N, et al. A phase II comparative study of gross tumor volume definition with or without PET/CT fusion in dosimetric planning for non-small-cell lung cancer (NSCLC): primary analysis of Radiation Therapy Oncology Group (RTOG)

0515. Int J Radiat Oncol Biol Phys 2012;82: 435–441 e1.

51. De Ruysscher D, Wanders S, Minken A, et al. Effects of radiotherapy planning with a dedicated combined PET-CT-simulator of patients with non-small cell lung cancer on dose limiting normal tissues and radiation dose-escalation: a planning study. Radiother Oncol 2005;77:5–10.

52. Faria SL, Menard S, Devic S, et al. Impact of FDG-PET/CT on radiotherapy volume delineation in non-small-cell lung cancer and correlation of imaging stage with pathologic findings. Int J Radiat Oncol Biol Phys 2008;70:1035–8.

53. Grills IS, Yan D, Black QC, et al. Clinical implications of defining the gross tumor volume with combination of CT and 18FDG-positron emission tomography in non-small-cell lung cancer. Int J Radiat Oncol Biol Phys 2007;67:709–19.

54. Macmanus M, D'Costa I, Everitt S, et al. Comparison of CT and positron emission tomography/CT coregistered images in planning radical radiotherapy in patients with non-small-cell lung cancer. Australas Radiol 2007;51:386–93.

55. Vinod SK, Kumar S, Holloway LC, et al. Dosimetric implications of the addition of 18 fluorodeoxyglucose-positron emission tomography in CT-based radiotherapy planning for non-small-cell lung cancer. J Med Imaging Radiat Oncol 2010;54:152–60.

56. Gondi V, Bradley K, Mehta M, et al. Impact of hybrid fluorodeoxyglucose positron-emission tomography/computed tomography on radiotherapy planning in esophageal and non-small-cell lung cancer. Int J Radiat Oncol Biol Phys 2007;67:187–95.

57. Kruser TJ, Bradley KA, Bentzen SM, et al. The impact of hybrid PET-CT scan on overall oncologic management, with a focus on radiotherapy planning: a prospective, blinded study. Technol Cancer Res Treat 2009;8:149–58.

58. Hanna GG, McAleese J, Carson KJ, et al. 18)F-FDG PET-CT simulation for non-small-cell lung cancer: effect in patients already staged by PET-CT. Int J Radiat Oncol Biol Phys 2010;77:24–30.

59. Yaremko B, Riauka T, Robinson D, et al. Threshold modification for tumour imaging in non-small-cell lung cancer using positron emission tomography. Nucl Med Commun 2005;26:433–40.

60. Moussallem M, Valette PJ, Traverse-Glehen A, et al. New strategy for automatic tumor segmentation by adaptive thresholding on PET/CT images. J Appl Clin Med Phys 2012;13:3875.

61. Turner LM, Howard JA, Dehghanpour P, et al. Exploring the feasibility of dose escalation positron emission tomography-positive disease with intensity-modulated radiation therapy and the effects on normal tissue structures for thoracic malignancies. Med Dosim 2011;36:383–8.

62. Wanet M, Delor A, Hanin FX, et al. An individualized radiation dose escalation trial in non-small cell lung cancer based on FDG-PET imaging. Strahlenther Onkol 2017;193:812–22.

63. Ohri N, Bodner WR, Kabarriti R, et al. Positron emission tomography-adjusted intensity modulated radiation therapy for locally advanced non-small cell lung cancer. Int J Radiat Oncol Biol Phys 2018;102:709–15.

64. Kong FM, Ten Haken RK, Schipper M, et al. Effect of midtreatment PET/CT-adapted radiation therapy with concurrent chemotherapy in patients with locally advanced non-small-cell lung cancer: a phase 2 clinical trial. JAMA Oncol 2017;3:1358–65.

65. Fried DV, Mawlawi O, Zhang L, et al. Potential use of (18)F-fluorodeoxyglucose positron emission tomography-based quantitative imaging features for guiding dose escalation in stage III non-small cell lung cancer. Int J Radiat Oncol Biol Phys 2016;94:368–76.

Diagnosis, Staging, Radiation Treatment Response Assessment, and Outcome Prognostication of Head and Neck Cancers Using PET Imaging: A Systematic Review

Nicole A. Hohenstein, BA[a], Jason W. Chan, MD[a], Susan Y. Wu, MD[a],
Peggy Tahir, MA, MLIS[b], Sue S. Yom, MD, PhD, MAS[a,*]

KEYWORDS

- PET/CT • Diagnosis • Staging • Radiation treatment response • Outcome prognostication
- Head and neck cancer • Hypoxia • Systematic review

KEY POINTS

- Diagnosis: ^{18}F-FDG PET/CT is recommended before pan-endoscopy or other invasive procedures in the workup for head and neck squamous cell carcinoma (HNSCC) of unknown primary.
- Staging: ^{18}F-FDG PET/CT is recommended in patients with locoregionally advanced HNSCC given its high level of accuracy in detecting nodal disease and sensitivity for distant metastases.
- Radiation treatment response: ^{18}F-FDG PET/CT at 12 weeks after completion of definitive chemo-radiation negates the need for planned neck dissection in up to 80% of cases without compromising overall survival.
- Outcome prognostication: PET tracers of hypoxia are promising prognostic biomarkers in HNSCC that merit further validation.

INTRODUCTION

[18F]Fluorodeoxyglucose (^{18}F-FDG) PET/computed tomography (CT) imaging has become an indispensable tool in all phases of oncologic management and is particularly useful for head and neck malignancies. In cases of head and neck cancer of unknown primary origin, ^{18}F-FDG PET/CT increases the likelihood of identifying the primary tumor and establishing the diagnosis. Furthermore, ^{18}F-FDG PET/CT is important in the accurate staging of locally advanced cases of head and neck squamous cell carcinoma (HNSCC), which can greatly affect recommendations for treatment. Following definitive chemoradiation, ^{18}F-FDG PET/CT is validated as a means of treatment response assessment and negates the need for planned neck dissection in most cases. Several hypoxia PET tracers have been studied in the context of radiotherapy dose escalation and prognostication.

Disclosure Statement: The authors have no relevant financial or commercial interests to disclose.
[a] Department of Radiation Oncology, Helen Diller Comprehensive Cancer Care Center, University of California San Francisco, 1600 Divisadero Street, Suite H-1031, San Francisco, CA 94143-1708, USA; [b] UCSF Radiation Oncology, UCSF Library, University of California San Francisco, 530 Parnassus Ave, San Francisco, CA 94143, USA
* Corresponding author.
E-mail address: sue.yom@ucsf.edu

PET Clin 15 (2020) 65–75
https://doi.org/10.1016/j.cpet.2019.08.010
1556-8598/20/© 2019 The Authors. Published by Elsevier Inc. This is an open access article under the CC BY-NC-ND license (http://creativecommons.org/licenses/by-nc-nd/4.0/).

METHODS

A comprehensive literature search was conducted to inform this summary of evidence-based practices related to PET/CT in head and neck cancer. The search included articles published from first occurrence of the search syntax through the end date of March 31, 2019 on EMBASE, Web of Science, and PubMed. Search terms were: head and/or neck cancer and PET/CT, with either staging, nodal sensitivity, postradiation assessment, or hypoxia tracer. Case reports or poster/presentation abstracts were automatically excluded. Titles and abstracts of the searched articles were initially screened for topical relevance and originality of scientific contribution, eliminating a large number of unrelated or noncontributory abstracts. To this remaining group of abstracts, 24 additional abstracts were added from other sources including expert opinion and citations from additional high-impact publications found through the literature search. The abstracts were then classified into 4 major groups, namely diagnosis, staging, radiation treatment response, and prognostication, and at least 2 postgraduate physicians were assigned to each group to review the data in more detail. After additional removal of unrelated, nonoriginal, or noncontributory material, the final set of selected abstracts was used to form the evidence basis of this review. See **Fig. 1** for more details.

DIAGNOSIS
Head and Neck Squamous Cell Carcinomas of Unknown Primary

Head and neck squamous cell carcinomas of unknown primary (HNSCCUP) make up 3% to 5% of all head and neck cancers. ^{18}F-FDG PET/CT is part of the standard workup for HNSCCUP and generally should be performed before pan-endoscopy and/or biopsies that may lead to false-positive findings on ^{18}F-FDG PET/CT. Primary tumor detection rates attributable to inclusion of ^{18}F-FDG PET/CT in the workup of HNSCCUP are summarized in **Table 1**.

Postreconstruction Tumor Persistence or Recurrence

Following regional or free-flap reconstruction, tumor persistence and/or recurrence is difficult to detect by physical examination alone. Post-treatment changes along the perimeter of the flap are difficult to distinguish from the tumor using cross-sectional imaging alone. The addition of ^{18}F-FDG PET to cross-sectional imaging improves the specificity of identifying tumor persistence or recurrence over contrast-enhanced cross-sectional imaging alone (**Table 2**).

Thyroid Incidentalomas

^{18}F-FDG-avid thyroid lesions incidentally discovered on whole-body ^{18}F-FDG PET/CT scans, or "incidentalomas," may lead to a diagnosis of thyroid cancer. The prevalence of incidentalomas is 1% to 3% and roughly one-third of these lesions are expected to be malignant; thus, all thyroid nodules with ^{18}F-FDG uptake should undergo biopsy (**Table 3**). Furthermore, the level of ^{18}F-FDG uptake provides insight into the histology of the thyroid carcinoma (**Table 4**). Well-differentiated thyroid carcinomas have high ^{131}I uptake and poor ^{18}F-FDG uptake. Conversely, poorly differentiated thyroid carcinomas—such as Hurthle cell carcinomas and anaplastic thyroid carcinomas— have poor ^{131}I uptake and more ^{18}F-FDG-avidity. ^{18}F-FDG PET is more sensitive in detecting lesions of medullary thyroid carcinoma when calcitonin exceeds 1000 ng/mL or carcinoembryonic antigen (CEA) exceeds 5 ng/mL.

STAGING
T Staging

^{18}F-FDG PET/CT is part of the standard workup of locoregionally advanced HNSCC because it improves the accuracy of nodal staging and detects more distant lesions than cross-sectional imaging alone. However, for the purpose of T-stage designation, ^{18}F-FDG PET/CT generally offers no improvement over conventional CT and/or MRI alone (**Table 5**) with the exception of oral cavity cancer in patients with dental artifact.[17] Roh and colleagues[13] compared the diagnostic utility of ^{18}F-FDG PET/CT with ^{18}F-FDG PET alone or CT/MRI in 167 patients with newly diagnosed HNSCC. In the detection of primary tumors, the researchers found that ^{18}F-FDG PET alone had a sensitivity of 98%, ^{18}F-FDG PET/CT had a sensitivity of 97%, and CT/MRI had a sensitivity of 86% to 88%. Although ^{18}F-FDG PET/CT offers higher sensitivity compared with CT/MRI, the investigators note that ^{18}F-FDG PET/CT does not provide enough anatomic depth and surrounding structure detail necessary for surgical planning for primary tumor resection, so that CT/MRI is still required. Seitz and colleagues[14] evaluated the impact of combined ^{18}F-FDG PET/CT versus MRI alone for T and N staging of 66 patients with oral and

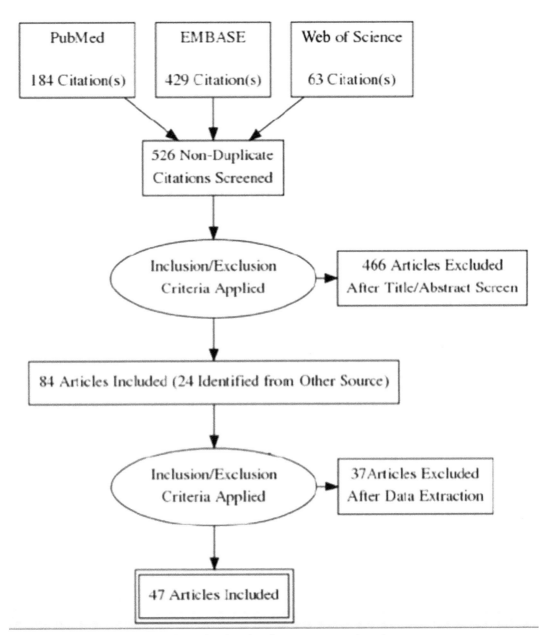

Fig. 1. PRISMA diagram: PET/CT utility in head and neck cancer systematic review.

oropharyngeal cancer. For primary tumors, ^{18}F-FDG PET/CT had a sensitivity of 96.7% and a specificity of 60%, whereas MRI had a sensitivity of 100% and a specificity of 80%. Seitz and colleagues[14] found no statistical difference between ^{18}F-FDG PET/CT and MRI in detecting primary disease ($P \geq .72$). Both imaging modalities had 100% sensitivity for detecting recurrent lesions. These investigators concluded that ^{18}F-FDG PET/CT and MRI have similar detection for primary tumors, and ^{18}F-FDG PET/CT is not

a superior imaging modality for staging primary tumors.

N Staging

By contrast, most studies show that the sensitivity of CT and/or MRI alone in detecting nodal involvement is relatively poor and ^{18}F-FDG PET significantly outperforms cross-sectional imaging in identifying malignant nodes (**Table 6**). Nguyen and colleagues[18] conducted a retrospective

Table 1
Diagnostic utility of ^{18}F-FDG PET/CT for head and neck squamous cell carcinoma of unknown primary

Study, Year	Design	Primary Detection Rate (%)	Sensitivity (%)	Specificity (%)
Rusthoven et al,[1] 2004	Systematic review of 16 studies (1994–2003)	74 of 302 (25)	88	75
Johansen et al,[2] 2008	Prospective	18 of 60 (30)	87	68
Rudmik et al,[3] 2011	Prospective	11 of 20 (55)	95	62
Lee et al,[4] 2015	Prospective	31 of 56 (55)	69	88

review of 71 patients with HNSCC who underwent MRI or CT and ^{18}F-FDG PET/CT before neck dissection. They found that both CT or MRI alone and ^{18}F-FDG PET/CT statistically correlated with pathologic findings ($P = .0001$; $P = .0001$), but ^{18}F-FDG PET/CT had a statistically higher prediction of true pathologic disease compared with CT or MRI alone for primary disease and nodal disease ($P = .005$ and $P = .013$, respectively). In detecting cervical lymph nodes as confirmed by pathologic staging, ^{18}F-FDG PET/CT had sensitivity of 94.5%, specificity of 89.9%, PPV (positive predictive value) of 90.8%, and NPV (negative predictive value) of 93.9%, whereas CT or MRI alone had sensitivity of 79.4%, specificity of 89.9%, PPV of 89.2%, and NPV of 80.5%. ^{18}F-FDG PET/CT was more reliable at identifying positive disease compared with CT or MRI alone ($P = .005$). Therefore, the authors recommend the use of ^{18}F-FDG PET/CT over CT or MRI alone when assessing cervical lymph node metastases.

Park and colleagues[20] conducted a prospective study of 160 patients with HNSCC using histopathology from neck dissections as the reference standard, finding that 58.8% (94/160) of patients had neck metastasis in 973 levels and 20 patients (21.3%) had contralateral neck metastasis. The researchers found that in per-patient, per-side, and per-level analyses, ^{18}F-FDG PET/CT was more sensitive than CT/MRI (91.5% vs 73.4%, $P<.001$; 91.1% vs 69.6%, $P<.001$; 91.1% vs 53%, $P<.001$, respectively). Additionally, for contralateral neck metastasis, ^{18}F-FDG PET/CT was more sensitive and accurate than CT/MRI (85.0% vs 45%, $P = .008$; 91.6% vs 80.3%, $P = .008$, respectively). Fleming and colleagues[22] found that in 67 patients who underwent ^{18}F-FDG PET/CT before neck dissection for nodal metastasis, ^{18}F-FDG PET/CT had a PPV of 92.7% and in 20 patients undergoing bilateral neck dissection, the accuracy of ^{18}F-FDG PET/CT was 89.7%. Owing to the high PPV, the investigators recommend imaging patients newly diagnosed with head and neck cancer with ^{18}F-FDG PET/CT to detect lymph node metastases.

M Staging

Furthermore, ^{18}F-FDG PET increases the sensitivity and specificity when added to CT or MRI in detecting distant metastases (**Table 7**). For distant metastases, Chan and colleagues[21] found that ^{18}F-FDG PET/MRI had a sensitivity of 90% and a PPV of 93.1%, whole-body MRI had a sensitivity of 86.7% with a PPV of 78.88%, and ^{18}F-FDG PET/CT had a sensitivity of 83.3% and a PPV of 83.3%. For bone metastases ^{18}F-FDG PET/MRI had a higher PPV (100%) compared with ^{18}F-FDG PET/CT (81.8%). Furthermore, Chan

Table 2
Diagnostic utility of ^{18}F-FDG PET/CT following reconstructive surgery

Study, Year	Design	n	Surveillance Technique	Sensitivity (%)	Specificity (%)
Oliver et al,[5] 2008	Retrospective	11	PET/CT	88	86
Müller et al,[6] 2015	Retrospective	27	PET/CT	88	79–89
			CT	75–88	68–79

Table 3
Systematic reviews of ^{18}F-FDG PET–detected thyroid incidentalomas

Study, Year	No. of Studies; No. of Patients	Prevalence of Incidentalomas (%)	Proportion of Incidentalomas that Are Malignant (%)	Mean SUV$_{max}$ for Malignant Lesions
Shie et al,[7] 2009	18; 55160 (1998–2007)	1.0	33	6.8 ± 4.6
Bertagna et al,[8] 2012	27; 147505 (no start date until 2012)	2.5	33–38	No reliable SUV cutoff

and colleagues[24] conducted a prospective study of 103 patients with untreated oropharyngeal or hypopharyngeal SCC. Eighteen (17.5%) of the patients had either a distant metastasis or a second primary cancer. On a per-lesion basis, ^{18}F-FDG PET/CT had a higher sensitivity (81.0%) than whole-body MRI (61.9%) ($P = .125$). Kao and colleagues[23] conducted a retrospective cohort study looking at the role of ^{18}F-FDG PET/CT within 6 months after radiation therapy in patients with head and/or neck cancer. The researchers found that for secondary tumor sites or distant metastases, ^{18}F-FDG PET/CT offered a sensitivity of 93%, a specificity of 96%, a PPV of 81%, and an NPV of 98%.

RADIATION TREATMENT RESPONSE ASSESSMENT

^{18}F-FDG PET/CT has become an important aspect of the postradiation response assessment.[25] ^{18}F-FDG PET/CT at 12 to 16 weeks after definitive chemoradiation in locally advanced HNSCC has been shown to have an NPV of greater than 90%, and planned neck dissection can be deferred in cases of radiographic complete treatment response.[26] Mehanna and colleagues[27] reported a randomized controlled trial ("PET-NECK") that tested the noninferiority of a surveillance ^{18}F-FDG PET/CT

performed 12 weeks after definitive chemoradiation versus planned neck dissection in mostly N2 and a few N3 (3%) HNSCCs. Patients who had a complete response at the primary site but an incomplete or equivocal response in the neck underwent neck dissection 4 weeks after ^{18}F-FDG PET/CT. The 2-year overall survival was similar in the 2 arms (85% and 82%) but 80% fewer neck dissections were performed with ^{18}F-FDG PET/CT surveillance, resulting in overall cost savings. This can also allow for less patient morbidity. However, it should be noted that ^{18}F-FDG PET/CT has a low PPV because there are high rates of false positives that often lead to additional imaging and unnecessary biopsies[28,29] and neck dissections in individual cases.

PROGNOSTICATION
[^{18}F]Fluoromisonidazole PET/Computed Tomography

Tumor hypoxia has been shown to correlate with worse treatment outcomes and is thought to be a major driver in treatment resistance as well as carrying a poor prognosis for patients.[30,31] Hypoxia has been shown to trigger angiogenesis, increase radioresistance, and reduce the effectiveness of surgery.[32] Polarographic electrodes were the first method used to measure

Table 4
Sensitivity of ^{18}F-FDG PET in detecting thyroid carcinomas

Study, Year	Population	Sensitivity (%)	Specificity (%)
Leboulleux et al,[9] 2007	^{18}F-FDG PET/CT	83	84
Riemann et al,[10] 2013	^{18}F-FDG PET/CT ^{131}I-WBS	92 65	95 94
Treglia et al,[11] 2012	Medullary thyroid carcinoma (MTC): calcitonin <150; ≥1000 ng/mL MTC: CEA <5; ≥5 ng/mL	40; 75 45; 69	—
Poisson et al,[12] 2010	Anaplastic thyroid carcinoma	62	—

Table 5
T-staging utility of ^{18}F-FDG PET/CT for head and neck squamous cell carcinomas

Study, Year	Design	n	Comparison	T-Stage Accuracy (%)* or Sensitivity (%)	
				PET	Comparison
Roh et al,[13] 2007	Retrospective	167	CT/MRI	97–98*	86–88*
Seitz et al,[14] 2009	Retrospective	66	MRI	97	100
Kanda et al,[15] 2013	Retrospective	30	MRI	67–87*	90*
Chaput et al,[16] 2018	Retrospective	35	MRI	83	63

tumor hypoxia, but this invasive technique was limited logistically and technically and was not recommended for widespread clinical use.[33] [^{18}F]Fluoromisonidazole (^{18}F-FMISO) PET/CT was the first hypoxia tracer introduced and has therefore been studied the most (**Table 8**).[32,35,39,40,44,45] ^{18}F-FMISO PET/CT has limitations including slow cellular washout in nonhypoxic tissue, which could lead to false positives, but also has a relatively short half-life that limits the amount of time available to wait for cellular washout.[35] Previous pattern-of-failure studies using ^{18}F-FMISO PET/CT have suggested that up to 50% of locoregional failures in HNSCCs occur because of hypoxia.[39] Löck and colleagues[30] showed that residual tumor hypoxia demonstrated by ^{18}F-FMISO PET/CT is associated with treatment resistance in HNSCC. The investigators recommended that hypoxia measured by^{18}F-FMISO PET/CT after week 2 of radiation treatment should identify patients who are at high risk of locoregional failure from chemoradiation. Lee and colleagues[34] assessed ^{18}F-FMISO uptake based on ^{18}F-FDG PET/CT gross tumor volume (GTV), and high areas of ^{18}F-FMISO uptake were targeted for a boost using intensity-

modulated radiation therapy (IMRT). Pigorsch and colleagues[46] studied whether dose escalation to the GTV would improve 2-year locoregional control and overall survival. This ESCALOC trial, a prospective randomized phase III trial, used cisplatin chemotherapy and an IMRT-based simultaneous integrated boost for patients with locoregionally advanced HNSCC. The total dose escalation to GTV was up to 80.5 Gy to the primary tumor and lymph nodes >2 cm. These investigators expect a 15% locoregional control benefit at 2 years.

^{18}F-HX4 PET/Computed Tomography

^{18}F-HX4 is a hydrophilic variant of the 2-nitroimidazole class of radiotracers that includes ^{18}F-FMISO and may offer a faster clearance time, and can theoretically distinguish between necrotic-hypoxic false-negative regions and viable hypoxic tumor cells.[31] Betts and colleagues[31] evaluated tumor hypoxia of the primary tumor in 3 patients with newly diagnosed HNSCC using ^{18}F-HX4 PET/CT scanning before definitive chemoradiation. The level of ^{18}F-HX4 tumor uptake varied between patients, suggesting a difference

Table 6
N-staging utility of ^{18}F-FDG PET/CT for head and neck squamous cell carcinomas

Study, Year	Design	n	Comparison	N-Stage Accuracy (%)* or Sensitivity (%)		N-Stage Specificity (%)	
				PET	Comparison	PET	Comparison
Roh et al,[13] 2007	Retrospective	167	CT/MRI	89	79	—	—
Seitz et al,[14] 2009	Retrospective	66	MRI	84	74	—	—
Kanda et al,[15] 2013	Retrospective	30	MRI	77*	63*	—	—
Nguyen et al,[18] 2013	Retrospective	71	CT/MRI	95	79	90	90
Roh et al,[19] 2014	Prospective	91	CT/MRI	71	50	81	87
Park et al,[20] 2016	Prospective	160	CT/MRI	92	73	—	—
Chan et al,[21] 2018	Retrospective	113	WB MRI	100	94	—	—

Table 7
M-staging utility of ^{18}F-FDG PET/CT for head and neck squamous cell carcinomas

Study, Year	Design	n	Comparison	M-Stage Sensitivity (%)		M-Stage Specificity (%)	
				PET	Comparison	PET	Comparison
Kao et al,[23] 2009	Retrospective	240	None	93	—	96	—
Chan et al,[24] 2011	Prospective	103	WB MRI	81	62	—	—
Kanda et al,[15] 2013	Retrospective	30	MRI	77	46	96	99
Chan et al,[21] 2018	Retrospective	113	WB MRI	90	87	—	—

in oxygenation profiles between histologically similar tumors.

^{18}F-FX4 PET/Computed Tomography

Thirty-two patients with HNSCC underwent ^{18}F-FX4 PET/CT at baseline and after approximately 20 Gy, in addition to blood hypoxia marker monitoring with carbonic anhydrase IX (CAIX), plasma osteopontin, and vascular endothelial growth factor (VEGF).[38] At baseline, tumor hypoxia was detected in 69% (22 of 32 patients) of the GTVs. The hypoxic fraction (HF) decreased from 21.7% ± 19.8% (baseline) to 3.6% ± 10.0% (during treatment) ($P<.001$). Although the researchers observed marked changes in hypoxia from the ^{18}F-FX4 PET/CT, there were no significant changes in CAIX and VEGF during treatment.[38] Concentrations of osteopontin did weakly correlate with the mean standardized uptake value (SUV_{mean}) of ^{18}F-FX4 PET/CT ($R = 0.52$, $P = .03$). Hypoxia PET/CT tracers may offer more sensitivity in monitoring changes in tissue hypoxia throughout treatment compared with blood markers.

^{18}F-EF5 PET/Computed Tomography

Komar and colleagues[33] used ^{18}F-EF5 PET imaging to assess tumor hypoxia in HNSCC patients. The researchers also evaluated tumor blood flow with the perfusion tracer ^{15}O-H$_2$O. Fifteen patients with 13 primary tumors and 5 lymph node metastases were included in the study. A voxel-to-voxel analysis found that all regions with high blood flow as measured by the ^{15}O-H$_2$O tracer had an ^{18}F-EF5 tumor-to-muscle ratio (T/M) of less than 1.5, and there was a positive correlation between blood flow and T/M ($r = 0.621$, $P<.0001$). By contrast, areas with minimal blood blow (<30 mL/100 g/min) showed a negative correlation between blood flow and T/M ($r = -0.042$, $P = .259$). Importantly, blood flow and hypoxia decreased and increased, respectively, at approximately the same rate ($r = 0.295$, $P<.0001$). In the first human study of ^{18}F-EF5 PET hypoxia marker, Komar and colleagues[33] observed that ^{18}F-EF5 accurately indicated hypoxia on PET imaging, had uniform access to all tissues, and was excreted primarily via the kidneys with no detectable metabolism. The researchers proposed a 3-h time point as the optimal time for detecting hypoxia-specific binding for head and neck cancer and a T/M threshold of 1.5 to determine the presence of hypoxia using ^{18}F-EF5.

Komar and colleagues[47] determined the predictive value for overall survival of pretreatment PET/CT imaging using ^{18}F-FDG, ^{18}F-EF5, and ^{15}O-H$_2$O in 22 patients with HNSCC treated with chemoradiation. Parametric blood flow was calculated using dynamic ^{15}O-H$_2$O PET images using a 1-tissue compartment while the metabolic activity of tumors and SUV was calculated based on ^{18}F-FDG images. T/M uptake ratios were calculated based on ^{18}F-EF5 images, and a T/M ratio of 1.5 was considered a significant threshold in determining tumor hypoxia subvolumes. Komar and colleagues[47] found a shorter overall survival with metabolically active tumor volume ($P = .008$, hazard ratio [HR] 1.108), maximum ^{18}F-EF5 T/M ratio ($P = .0145$, HR 4.084), and tumor hypoxia subvolumes ($P = .0047$ HR 1.112). There were no statistically significant correlations among ^{18}F-FDG SUV_{max}, ^{18}F-EF5 T/M ratio, and blood flow. Compared with ^{18}F-FDG uptake, high uptake of the hypoxia tracer ^{18}F-EF5 was strongly correlated with poor clinical outcomes.

[^{18}F]-Fluoroazomycin Arabinoside PET/Computed Tomography

Servagi-Vernat and colleagues[37] imaged 12 patients with locally advanced HNSCC with [^{18}F]fluoroazomycin arabinoside (^{18}F-FAZA) PET/CT before treatment, after 7 fractions, and after 17 fractions of definitive chemoradiation. Ten of the 12 patients had hypoxic volumes identified

Table 8
Select hypoxia tracer studies in head and neck squamous cell carcinomas

Study, Year	n	Tracer	Significance
Lee et al,[34] 2008	10	^{18}F-FMISO	Assessed ^{18}F-FMISO uptake based on ^{18}F-FDG PET/CT GTV and high areas of ^{18}F-FMISO uptake were target for an IMRT boost. The areas of hypoxia received 84 Gy and GTV received 70 Gy
Komar et al,[33] 2008	15	^{18}F-EF5	^{18}F-EF5 accurately indicated hypoxia on PET imaging
Choi et al,[35] 2010	8	^{18}F-FMISO	Defined hypoxic tumor volume using a tumor-to-cerebellum ratio (T/C) of 1.3 as the threshold for ^{18}F-FMISO PET/CT
Lanning et al,[36] 2014	21	^{18}F-FMISO	Of the 13 patients with nodal hypoxia on original scan, 6 underwent dose de-escalation at the indexed lymph node. IMRT dose de-escalation demonstrated no clinical evidence of disease or unremarkable treatment toxicity at 3-mo follow-up
Servagi-Vernat et al,[37] 2015	12	^{18}F-FAZA	Successfully dose-escalated areas found to be hypoxic with ^{18}F-FAZA PET/CT to 86 Gy
Zegers et al,[38] 2016	32	^{18}F-HX4	Detected tumor hypoxia in 69% (22 of 32 patients) of the GTVs. HF decrease from 21.7% $\pm$ 19.8% (baseline) to 3.6% $\pm$ 10.0% (during treatment) ($P<.001$)
Boeke et al,[39] 2017	54	^{18}F-FMISO	Compared the pretherapeutic hypoxic subvolumes detected by ^{18}F-FMISO PET/CT with the spatial location of failures using CT or ^{18}F-FDG PET/CT
Crispin-Ortuzar et al,[32] 2017	75	^{18}F-FMISO	Propose that ^{18}F-FDG PET/CT could be a viable alternative to detect hypoxia if ^{18}F-FMISO PET/CT is unavailable
Grkovski et al,[40] 2017	75	^{18}F-FMISO	Found that ^{18}F-FMISO PET dynamic imaging revealed more detail on tumor microenvironment and assessment of chemoradiation response compared with a single static image based on pharmacokinetic modeling
Welz et al,[41] 2017	25	^{18}F-FMISO	10 patients randomized to dose-escalated 77 Gy/35 fractions to hypoxic regions. 2-y locoregional control was significantly worse in the patients with hypoxia who received standard chemoradiation compared with the nonhypoxia tumor patients who received standard chemoradiation (44.4% vs 100%, $P = .048$)
Suh et al,[42] 2017	15	^{64}Cu-ATSM	Identified 16 genes that were positively associated and 5 genes that were negatively associated with hypoxia volume (adjusted $P<.1$; 8 genes had adjusted $P<.05$; hypoxic volume-associated gene signature)
Betts et al,[31] 2019	3	^{18}F-HX4	Evaluated tumor hypoxia of the primary tumor in a small series of patients (3) with newly diagnosed HNSCC using ^{18}F-HX4 PET/CT scan before chemoradiation
Bandurska-Luque et al,[43] 2019	45	^{18}F-FMISO	Found that bigger lymph node metastases had similar hypoxia levels compared with primary tumors while smaller lymph node metastases were less hypoxic
Löck et al,[30] 2019	50	^{18}F-FMISO	58 hypoxia-associated genes were correlated with tumor-to-background ratio and hypoxic volume

by ^{18}F-FAZA PET/CT. After the second scan, 7 patients had a previously nonhypoxic, newborn hypoxic voxel that appeared in the primary tumor and/or a lymph node. After the third scan, only 3 patients still had newborn voxels. Treatment planning occurred in three phases after each

^{18}F-FAZA PET/CT scan, with the goal of delivering a fixed dose of 86 Gy to any voxels defined as hypoxic. ^{18}F-FAZA PET/CT-detected hypoxic regions were dose-escalated without substantial dose increase to surrounding tissues. The researchers found that implementing hypoxia-

tracing scans before and during treatment allowed them to plan in multiple phases and adapt to changes in hypoxia status over time.

[^{64}Cu]Diacetyl-bis(N-Methylthiosemicarbazone) PET/Computed Tomography

Suh and colleagues[42] compared hypoxia biomarkers and gene expression in oropharyngeal SCC diagnostic biopsies using [^{64}Cu]diacetyl-bis(N-methylthiosemicarbazone) (^{64}Cu-ATSM) PET/CT hypoxia tracer imaging. Using a cohort of 15 patients, the authors identified 16 genes that were positively associated and 5 genes that were negatively associated with hypoxia volume (adjusted $P<.1$; 8 genes had adjusted $P<.05$; hypoxic volume-associated gene signature). In addition, a 21-gene signature was associated with inferior 3-year progression-free survival (HR 1.5 (1.0–2.2), $P = .047$).

SUMMARY

In summary, ^{18}F-FDG PET is a tool in the diagnosis, staging, and radiation treatment response assessment of head and neck cancers that is supported by substantial evidence. In cases of HNSCCUP, the addition of ^{18}F-FDG PET to cross-sectional imaging increases the likelihood of identifying the primary site. In thyroid incidentalomas, ^{18}F-FDG avidity raises the suspicion of malignancy and can lead to the diagnosis of thyroid cancers. Furthermore, ^{18}F-FDG PET is a useful staging tool, particularly in the nodal and distant metastatic assessment of HNSCC. Post-treatment response assessment with ^{18}F-FDG PET is recommended at roughly 12 weeks for HNSCCs. Finally, many non-^{18}F-FDG tracers that reflect hypoxia, proliferation, and metabolism are actively being studied and have promise in the prognostication of different cancer types and the targeting of resistant disease.

SUPPLEMENTARY DATA

Supplementary content related to this article can be found at https://doi.org/10.1016/j.cpet.2019.08.010.

REFERENCES

1. Rusthoven KE, Koshy M, Paulino AC. The role of fluorodeoxyglucose positron emission tomography in cervical lymph node metastases from an unknown primary tumor. Cancer 2004;101(11):2641–9.
2. Johansen J, Buus S, Loft A, et al. Prospective study of ^{18}FDG-PET in the detection and management of patients with lymph node metastases to the neck from an unknown primary tumor. Results from the DAHANCA-13 study. Head Neck 2008;30(4):471–8.
3. Rudmik L, Lau HY, Matthews TW, et al. Clinical utility of PET/CT in the evaluation of head and neck squamous cell carcinoma with an unknown primary: a prospective clinical trial. Head Neck 2011;33(7):935–40.
4. Lee JR, Kim JS, Roh J-L, et al. Detection of occult primary tumors in patients with cervical metastases of unknown primary tumors: comparison of (18)F FDG PET/CT with contrast-enhanced CT or CT/MR imaging-prospective study. Radiology 2015;274(3):764–71.
5. Oliver C, Muthukrishnan A, Mountz J, et al. Interpretability of PET/CT imaging in head and neck cancer patients following composite mandibular resection and osteocutaneous free flap reconstruction. Head Neck 2008;30(2):187–93.
6. Müller J, Hüllner M, Strobel K, et al. The value of (18)F-FDG-PET/CT imaging in oral cavity cancer patients following surgical reconstruction. Laryngoscope 2015;125(8):1861–8.
7. Shie P, Cardarelli R, Sprawls K, et al. Systematic review: prevalence of malignant incidental thyroid nodules identified on fluorine-18 fluorodeoxyglucose positron emission tomography. Nucl Med Commun 2009;30(9):742–8.
8. Bertagna F, Treglia G, Piccardo A, et al. Diagnostic and clinical significance of F-18-FDG-PET/CT thyroid incidentalomas. J Clin Endocrinol Metab 2012;97(11):3866–75.
9. Leboulleux S, Schroeder PR, Schlumberger M, et al. The role of PET in follow-up of patients treated for differentiated epithelial thyroid cancers. Nat Clin Pract Endocrinol Metab 2007;3(2):112–21.
10. Riemann B, Uhrhan K, Dietlein M, et al. Diagnostic value and therapeutic impact of (18)F-FDG-PET/CT in differentiated thyroid cancer. Results of a German multicentre study. Nuklearmedizin 2013;52(1):1–6.
11. Treglia G, Villani MF, Giordano A, et al. Detection rate of recurrent medullary thyroid carcinoma using fluorine-18 fluorodeoxyglucose positron emission tomography: a meta-analysis. Endocrine 2012;42(3):535–45.
12. Poisson T, Deandreis D, Leboulleux S, et al. ^{18}F-fluorodeoxyglucose positron emission tomography and computed tomography in anaplastic thyroid cancer. Eur J Nucl Med Mol Imaging 2010;37(12):2277–85.
13. Roh J-L, Yeo N-K, Kim JS, et al. Utility of 2-[^{18}F] fluoro-2-deoxy-D-glucose positron emission tomography and positron emission tomography/computed tomography imaging in the preoperative staging of head and neck squamous cell carcinoma. Oral Oncol 2007;43(9):887–93.
14. Seitz O, Chambron-Pinho N, Middendorp M, et al. ^{18}F-Fluorodeoxyglucose-PET/CT to evaluate tumor,

nodal disease, and gross tumor volume of oropha-
ryngeal and oral cavity cancer: comparison with
MR imaging and validation with surgical specimen.
Neuroradiology 2009;51(10):677–86.

15. Kanda T, Kitajima K, Suenaga Y, et al. Value of retrospective image fusion of ^{18}F-FDG PET and MRI for
preoperative staging of head and neck cancer:
comparison with PET/CT and contrast-enhanced
neck MRI. Eur J Radiol 2013;82(11):2005–10.

16. Chaput A, Robin P, Podeur F, et al. Diagnostic performance of [18]fluorodesoxyglucose positron emis-
sion/computed   tomography   and   magnetic
resonance imaging in detecting T1-T2 head and
neck squamous cell carcinoma. Laryngoscope
2018;128(2):378–85.

17. Baek C-H, Chung MK, Son Y-I, et al. Tumor volume
assessment by ^{18}F-FDG PET/CT in patients with
oral cavity cancer with dental artifacts on CT or MR
images. J Nucl Med 2008;49(9):1422–8.

18. Nguyen A, Luginbuhl A, Cognetti D, et al. Effectiveness of PET/CT in the preoperative evaluation
of neck disease. Laryngoscope 2014;124(1):
159–64.

19. Roh J-L, Park JP, Kim JS, et al. [18]F fluorodeoxyglucose PET/CT in head and neck squamous cell carcinoma with negative neck palpation findings: a
prospective study. Radiology 2014;271(1):153–61.

20. Park JT, Roh J-L, Kim JS, et al. (18)F FDG PET/CT
versus CT/MR imaging and the prognostic value of
contralateral neck metastases in patients with head
and neck squamous cell carcinoma. Radiology
2016;279(2):481–91.

21. Chan S-C, Yeh C-H, Yen T-C, et al. Clinical utility of
simultaneous whole-body ^{18}F-FDG PET/MRI as a
single-step imaging modality in the staging of primary nasopharyngeal carcinoma. Eur J Nucl Med
Mol Imaging 2018;45(8):1297–308.

22. Fleming AJ, Smith SP, Paul CM, et al. Impact of
[18]F]-2-fluorodeoxyglucose-positron emission to-
mography/computed tomography on previously untreated head and neck cancer patients.
Laryngoscope 2007;117(7):1173–9.

23. Kao J, Vu HL, Genden EM, et al. The diagnostic and
prognostic utility of positron emission tomography/
computed tomography-based follow-up after radiotherapy for head and neck cancer. Cancer 2009;
115(19):4586–94.

24. Chan S-C, Wang H-M, Yen T-C, et al. ^{18}F-FDG PET/
CT and 3.0-T whole-body MRI for the detection of
distant metastases and second primary tumours in
patients with untreated oropharyngeal/hypophar-
yngeal carcinoma: a comparative study. Eur J Nucl
Med Mol Imaging 2011;38(9):1607–19.

25. Connell CA, Corry J, Milner AD, et al. Clinical impact
of, and prognostic stratification by, F-18 FDG PET/
CT in head and neck mucosal squamous cell carcinoma. Head Neck 2007;29(11):986–95.

26. Helsen N, Van den Wyngaert T, Carp L, et al. FDG-
PET/CT for treatment response assessment in
head and neck squamous cell carcinoma: a systematic review and meta-analysis of diagnostic performance. Eur J Nucl Med Mol Imaging 2018;45(6):
1063–71.

27. Mehanna H, Wong W-L, McConkey CC, et al. PET-
CT surveillance versus neck dissection in advanced
head and neck cancer. N Engl J Med 2016;374(15):
1444–54.

28. Anderson CM, Chang T, Graham MM, et al. Change
of maximum standardized uptake value slope in dynamic triphasic ^{18}F]-fluorodeoxyglucose positron
emission tomography/computed tomography distin-
guishes malignancy from postradiation inflammation
in head-and-neck squamous cell carcinoma: a prospective trial. Int J Radiat Oncol Biol Phys 2015;
91(3):472–9.

29. Gupta T, Jain S, Agarwal JP, et al. Diagnostic performance of response assessment FDG-PET/CT in
patients with head and neck squamous cell carcinoma treated with high-precision definitive
(chemo)radiation. Radiother Oncol 2010;97(2):
194–9.

30. Löck S, Linge A, Seidlitz A, et al. Repeat FMISO-PET
imaging weakly correlates with hypoxia-associated
gene expressions for locally advanced HNSCC
treated by primary radiochemotherapy. Radiother
Oncol 2019;135:43–50.

31. Betts HM, O'Connor RA, Christian JA, et al. Hypoxia
imaging with ^{18}F]HX4 PET in squamous cell head
and neck cancers: a pilot study for integration into
treatment planning. Nucl Med Commun 2019;
40(1):73–8.

32. Crispin-Ortuzar M, Apte A, Grkovski M, et al. Predicting hypoxia status using a combination of
contrast-enhanced computed tomography and
[18]F]-fluorodeoxyglucose positron emission tomography radiomics features. Radiother Oncol 2018;
127(1):36–42.

33. Komar G, Seppänen M, Eskola O, et al. ^{18}F-EF5: a
new PET tracer for imaging hypoxia in head and
neck cancer. J Nucl Med 2008;49(12):1944–51.

34. Lee NY, Mechalakos JG, Nehmeh S, et al. Fluorine-
18-labeled fluoromisonidazole positron emission
and computed tomography-guided intensity-modulated radiotherapy for head and neck cancer: a
feasibility study. Int J Radiat Oncol Biol Phys 2008;
70(1):2–13.

35. Choi W, Lee S, Park SH, et al. Planning study for
available dose of hypoxic tumor volume using
fluorine-18-labeled fluoromisonidazole positron
emission tomography for treatment of the head
and neck cancer. Radiother Oncol 2010;97(2):
176–82.

36. Lanning RM, Beattie B, Humm J, et al. Preliminary
results of a prospective trial of IMRT dose de-

escalation to gross nodal disease in human papillo-mavirus (HPV)-Positive oropharyngeal carcinoma (OPC) based on assessment of tumor hypoxia using ^{18}F-FMISO pet imaging. Int J Radiat Oncol Biol Phys 2014;88(2):474.

37. Servagi-Vernat S, Differding S, Sterpin E, et al. Hypoxia-guided adaptive radiation dose escalation in head and neck carcinoma: a planning study. Acta Oncol 2015;54(7):1008–16.

38. Zegers CML, Hoebers FJP, van Elmpt W, et al. Evaluation of tumour hypoxia during radiotherapy using [F-18]HX4 PET imaging and blood biomarkers in patients with head and neck cancer. Eur J Nucl Med Mol Imaging 2016;43(12):2139–46.

39. Boeke S, Thorwarth D, Mönnich D, et al. Geometric analysis of loco-regional recurrences in relation to pre-treatment hypoxia in patients with head and neck cancer. Acta Oncol 2017;56(11):1571–6.

40. Grkovski M, Lee NY, Schöder H, et al. Monitoring early response to chemoradiotherapy with ^{18}F-FMISO dynamic PET in head and neck cancer. Eur J Nucl Med Mol Imaging 2017;44(10):1682–91.

41. Welz S, Mönnich D, Pfannenberg C, et al. Prognostic value of dynamic hypoxia PET in head and neck cancer: results from a planned interim analysis of a randomized phase II hypoxia-image guided dose escalation trial. Radiother Oncol 2017;124(3):526–32.

42. Suh Y-E, Lawler K, Henley-Smith R, et al. Association between hypoxic volume and underlying hypoxia-induced gene expression in oropharyngeal squamous cell carcinoma. Br J Cancer 2017;116(8):1057–64.

43. Bandurska-Luque A, Löck S, Haase R, et al. Correlation between FMISO-PET based hypoxia in the primary tumour and in lymph node metastases in locally advanced HNSCC patients. Clin Transl Radiat Oncol 2019;15:108–12.

44. Mammar H, Kerrou K, Nataf V, et al. Positron emission tomography/computed tomography imaging of residual skull base chordoma before radiotherapy using fluoromisonidazole and fluorodeoxyglucose: potential consequences for dose painting. Int J Radiat Oncol Biol Phys 2012;84(3):681–7.

45. Okamoto S, Shiga T, Yasuda K, et al. High reproducibility of tumor hypoxia evaluated by ^{18}F-fluoromisonidazole PET for head and neck cancer. J Nucl Med 2013;54(2):201–7.

46. Pigorsch SU, Wilkens JJ, Kampfer S, et al. Do selective radiation dose escalation and tumour hypoxia status impact the loco-regional tumour control after radio-chemotherapy of head & neck tumours? The ESCALOX protocol. Radiat Oncol 2017;12(1):45.

47. Komar G, Lehtiö K, Seppänen M, et al. Prognostic value of tumour blood flow, ^{18}F]EF5 and ^{18}F]FDG PET/CT imaging in patients with head and neck cancer treated with radiochemotherapy. Eur J Nucl Med Mol Imaging 2014;41(11):2042–50.

The Utility of PET/Computed Tomography for Radiation Oncology Planning, Surveillance, and Prognosis Prediction of Gastrointestinal Tumors

Stephanie R. Rice, MD[a], Michael Chuong, MD[b], Antony Koroulakis, MD[a], Osman M. Siddiqui, MD[a], Ankur M. Sharma, MD[c,d], Charles B. Simone II, MD[e], Jason K. Molitoris, MD, PhD[f], Adeel Kaiser, MD[f,*]

KEYWORDS

• PET/CT • Gastrointestinal • Staging • Prognosis

KEY POINTS

• At present, the strongest evidence for the use of PET/computed tomography (CT) in gastrointestinal (GI) malignancies is to rule out distant metastatic disease at diagnosis, radiation treatment planning for anal malignancies, and disease recurrence monitoring in colorectal and anal malignancies.
• Use of PET/CT for GI malignancies continues to evolve over time, with new studies evaluating prognostic abilities of PET/CT and with increasing sensitivity and spatial resolution of more modern PET/CT scanners.
• The authors encourage future applications and prospective evaluation of the use of PET/CT in the staging, prognostication, and recurrence prediction for GI malignancies.

INTRODUCTION

In 2018, gastrointestinal (GI) malignancies accounted for 26.3% and 18.6% of cancer diagnoses and 35.4% and 27.3% of cancer-related mortality worldwide and in the United States, respectively.[1–3] Staging work-up is critical for appropriate treatment selection in patients with cancer. The development of [^{18}F]-fluorodeoxyglucose (FDG) in PET dates back to the late 1970s,[4,5] and allowed a shift in the approach of imaging from anatomic to functional localization. The combination of PET/computed tomography (CT) became commercially available in 2001,[6] and allowed better anatomic localization of functional FDG uptake, with widespread use in the staging, treatment, prognostication, and surveillance of several malignancies. This article discusses the established uses of and emerging trends in PET/CT for staging, radiation

Disclosure Statement: Dr. Adeel Kaiser has a Speaker Agreement with Varian Medical Systems.
[a] Department of Radiation Oncology, University of Maryland Medical Center, 22 S. Greene Street, Baltimore, MD, USA; [b] Department of Radiation Oncology, Miami Cancer Institute, 8900 Kendall Drive, Miami, FL, USA; [c] Department of Radiation Oncology, Maryland Proton Treatment Center, University of Maryland School of Medicine, 850 West Baltimore Street, Baltimore, MD, USA; [d] Harvard T.H. Chan School of Public Health, Harvard University, 677 Huntington Avenue, Boston, MA, USA; [e] New York Proton Center, 225 East 126th Street, New York, NY, USA; [f] Department of Radiation Oncology, University of Maryland School of Medicine, 22 S. Greene Street, Baltimore, MD, USA
* Corresponding author.
E-mail address: akaiser@som.umaryland.edu

oncology treatment planning, prognostication, follow-up, and evaluation of recurrence of specific GI malignancies (**Table 1**).

ESOPHAGEAL CANCER
Initial Diagnosis and Staging

The National Comprehensive Cancer Network (NCCN) recommends staging work-up to include upper endoscopy with biopsy, contrast-enhanced CT scans of the chest and abdomen, endoscopic ultrasonography (EUS), and PET/CT.[7] A meta-analysis of EUS in staging showed a pooled sensitivity and specificity (sens/spec) of 81.6% to 91.4% and 94.4% to 99.4% for T1 to T3 lesions, and 92.4% and 97.4% for T4 lesions. The combination of EUS with fine-needle aspiration biopsy for nodal staging increases sensitivity from 84.7% to 96.7% and specificity from 84.6% to 95.5% versus EUS alone.[8]

A systematic review of PET/CT for locoregional staging showed lower sens/spec of 51% and 84%,[9] likely caused by obscuring of periesophageal lymph nodes in close proximity to the primary tumor, difficulty differentiating inflammatory processes from metastatic involvement, and/or presence of occult foci of metastatic disease that are below the threshold of PET/CT detection.[10]

At diagnosis, 20% to 30% of patients with esophageal cancer have metastatic disease. Lowe and colleagues[11] compared PET, EUS, and CT in the initial staging of 75 patients with esophageal cancer and found that the sens/spec was 81% and 91% for PET, 73% and 86% for EUS, and 81% and 82% for CT with a trend toward benefit favoring CT and PET. A meta-analysis assessing the utility of CT and PET/CT in the diagnosis of distant metastases found that the sens/spec for PET/CT was 71% and 93% versus 52% and 91% for CT.[12] Ultimately, several studies have shown a 20% distant metastases detection rate with PET/CT, suggesting a potential cost

benefit and avoidance of unnecessary esophagectomy.[13] A summary of sens/spec in staging across GI malignancy sites is provided in **Table 2**.

Treatment Planning, Postneoadjuvant Therapy, and Suspected Recurrence

Medically fit patients with locally advanced disease often undergo neoadjuvant therapy, and PET/CT has been shown to be helpful in aiding gross tumor volume (GTV) more accurately than CT when used in combination with EUS.[14] An example image of PET/CT GTV delineation is shown in **Fig. 1**. In addition, PET/CT may be beneficial in restaging before surgical resection to assess for interval development of metastatic disease. The Municon I study stratified patients based on response to chemotherapy to either receive surgery (nonresponders) or to continue 12 weeks of additional chemotherapy before surgery (responders), allowing early adaptive treatment based on individual tumor biology. The study showed an overall survival (OS) advantage in early responders compared with nonresponders (median OS not reached vs 25.8 months).[15] A retrospective analysis of 88 patients with potentially resectable esophageal cancer undergoing restaging PET/CT after neoadjuvant chemoradiation found interval metastases in 8% of cases.[16] A more recent meta-analysis and systematic review of 14 studies showed an 8% rate of true distant metastases after neoadjuvant treatment using FDG-PET/CT, but a 5% false-positive rate, suggesting that pathologic confirmation in this setting is warranted before deeming a patient as unresectable from metastatic disease.[17]

Following trimodality treatment, local anatomic changes can make interpretation of CT or endoscopic assessment difficult, and offers an opportunity for PET/CT as an adjunct. A systematic review of PET/CT for disease recurrence in esophageal cancer found a pooled sens/spec of 96%

Table 1
Recommendations for PET/computed tomography for gastrointestinal malignancies

Disease Site	Primary Work-up	RT Treatment Planning	Disease Response	Follow-up	Suspected Recurrence
Esophageal	A	PA	PA	I	PA
Gastric	PA	I	PA	PA	I
Hepatobiliary	PA	PA	I	I	I
Pancreatic	PA	PA	PA	I	PA
Colorectal	PA	PA	PA	PA	A
Anal	A	A	PA	I	A

Abbreviations: A, appropriate; I, inappropriate; PA, potentially appropriate; RT, radiation therapy.

Table 2
Sensitivity and specificity of PET/computed tomography in the primary work-up of gastrointestinal malignancies

Disease Site (Reference)	Sensitivity (%)	Specificity (%)
Esophageal[9–12]	51–81	84–93
Gastric[a,21–23]	58–98	33–86
Hepatobiliary[41–44]	55–96	79–88
Pancreatic[50–57]	89–91	71–88
Colorectal[78,81–83]	66–100	75–100
Anal[101,102]	93–100	53–87

[a] For lesions T2 or greater.

and 78%, respectively.[18] PET/CT may be most helpful in the setting of equivocal initial studies to differentiate recurrence from posttreatment change. At present, the NCCN guidelines list FDG-PET/CT as a potential surveillance option in patients with T1b disease after chemoradiation therapy; otherwise contrast-enhanced CT chest/abdomen and esophagogastroduodenoscopy are recommended.[7]

GASTRIC CANCER
Staging and Work-up

Staging work-up for the management of gastric cancer typically includes the use of upper GI endoscopy and biopsy, EUS, and contrast-enhanced CT of the chest, abdomen, and pelvis. In the setting of greater than T1 nonmetastatic disease, NCCN guidelines endorse the use of PET/CT in staging work-up.[19] In 1 study, the sensitivity of PET/CT for primary tumor detection was 93% to 98% for T2 or higher disease,[20] whereas another study showed locoregional sens/spec ranging from 58.3% to 83.0% and 85.7% to 95.2%.[21] Some of the wide variability is attributed to different histologies and tumor differentiation.[22,23] One study showed that by more accurately determining the true clinical stage of patients, the use of PET/CT in initial staging altered the overall treatment goal from neoadjuvant to palliative in

47.3% of patients.[24] Nodal staging with PET/CT affords good specificity (85.7%–97.0%), but low sensitivity (33.3%–64.6%),[22] and is most useful in detecting metastatic disease.[23,25–27] A recent retrospective study of 279 patients showed that routine PET/CT identifies unexpected metastases in 7.2% of patients, and that FDG-avid nodes had a higher likelihood of incurable disease,[28] supporting the use of PET/CT in staging of patients with gastric cancer. A summary of sens/spec in staging can be found in **Table 2**.

Prognostic Response to Therapy

Patients in a study who were undergoing preoperative chemotherapy were assigned to have PET/CT scans before chemotherapy and at 14 days after initiation of chemotherapy. Results from this study showed significantly increased histopathologic response (69%) and OS (median not reached) in patients with greater than 35% decrease in standardized uptake value (SUV).[29] It also showed that early salvage therapy in poor responders led to improvements in outcomes.[30] Although PET/CT for treatment adaptation and outcome prediction is not currently standard of care, this emerging evidence is intriguing and warrants further investigation in larger prospective trials.

Posttreatment and Surveillance

The NCCN guidelines do not recommend PET/CT for routine follow-up, but allow PET/CT in patients unable to undergo diagnostic CT imaging because of contrast allergy or renal insufficiency.[19] In the setting of disease recurrence, the same challenges of limited uptake depending on histology and tumor differentiation apply, and utility of PET/CT is uncertain in this scenario. A retrospective study of 33 patients with suspected recurrence showed that PET had a sens/spec of 70% and 69%, with positive and negative predictive values of 78% and 60%, respectively, and was therefore not recommended for follow-up imaging in gastric cancer. However, there was significantly improved survival in the PET-negative group.[31] Another retrospective study of disease

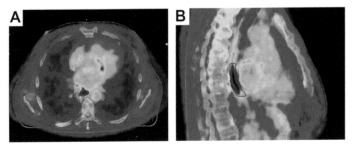

Fig. 1. PET from PET/CT performed for staging with outline of the GTV (*red contour*) for radiation treatment planning in the axial (*A*) and sagittal planes (*B*).

surveillance showed equivalent sens/spec between PET/CT and CT in all areas of recurrence except the peritoneum, where CT was more sensitive.[32] Because most of this evidence is based on small retrospective experiences, the recommendations of scientific societies vary.[19,33–35]

HEPATOBILIARY TUMORS

Abdominal multiphasic contrast-enhanced CT or magnetic resonance (MR) imaging remain the standard for staging of hepatobiliary tumors[36]; however, there may be a role for PET/CT when tumor is among biliary strictures and must be distinguished from benign disease. Researchers from Japan examined the utility of early and delayed PET imaging for biliary strictures, and found that delayed imaging (at 188 ± 27 minutes after FDG administration) showed greater SUV values in tumors than normal liver with sens/spec of 86% and 88%, respectively.[37] Data from Korea show a reduction in sensitivity of PET/CT imaging for perihilar lesions (83%) compared with intrahepatic (91%) and common bile duct cancers (91%).[38] PET/CT also improved the detection of occult regional nodal metastasis, which were biopsy confirmed, with a 77% concordance rate, compared with 31% with CT imaging alone.

Overall there is a lack of data regarding the utility of PET imaging to inform radiation treatment planning for hepatobiliary tumors.[39] However, 1 study from Turkey examined the impact of PET/CT on target volume delineation in 15 patients with unresectable extrahepatic cholangiocarcinoma (CC). The results showed a mean GTV volume reduction of 29% ($P = .008$) with the use of PET imaging.[40]

Hepatocellular Cancer

The utility of PET/CT as a diagnostic tool remains limited in hepatocellular carcinoma (HCC). Researchers from Saint Louis University examined the utility of PET versus CT imaging to distinguish between benign and malignant lesions in 20 patients with biopsy-proven disease, with a notable decrease in sensitivity of PET compared with CT (55% vs 90%) as well as decreased avidity among low-grade and well-differentiated tumors. However, PET did reveal metastases in 3 patients that were not seen on CT, suggesting that PET imaging may be useful in diagnosis and staging as an adjunct to CT for HCC.[41] A Japanese group compared the molecular mechanisms underlying the insufficient sensitivity of PET in HCC by comparing 14 metastatic colorectal cases with 20 patients with HCC.[42] Compared with metastases, HCC lesions showed lower hexokinase and glucose transporter 1 (GLUT1) expression as well

as higher expression of glucose-6-phosphatase. As an example, compared with surrounding liver tissue, GLUT1 overexpression was increased 92-fold in metastatic cases compared with only 11-fold in HCC. There was a dramatic difference between moderately and poorly differentiated HCC, with an average SUV of 4.0 ± 0.3 versus 14.4 ± 3.7 ($P<.0001$), respectively, suggesting a potential role for PET in poorly differentiated tumors.

Cholangiocarcinoma

In contrast with HCC, CC shows much greater sens/spec with diagnostic PET imaging. In a prospective study of 123 patients in Korea, PET scans showed sens/spec of 84% and 79%, with a positive predictive value of 93%.[43] PET also showed a superior ability compared with CT in distinguishing between regional nodal (76% vs 61%, $P = .004$) and distant (88% vs 79%, $P = .004$) metastases. This finding is corroborated by a study of 126 patients from Memorial Sloan Kettering Cancer Center in which 24% of patients with CC had staging and treatment plans altered by PET imaging.[44] Preoperative PET has also been shown to be a useful tool for predicting the likelihood of cancer recurrence after surgery. In a study of 357 patients with preoperative PET imaging for intrahepatic CC and HCC, maximum SUV was associated with both OS and early recurrence ($P<.05$).[45]

Gallbladder Cancer

Studies of PET/CT in gallbladder cancer support the use of this modality. Data from Memorial Sloan Kettering Cancer Center revealed a sensitivity of 78% for the detection of primary tumors and 96% for the detection of metastatic disease, with PET altering management in 23% of cases.[44] Similarly, data from Spain suggest a PET sens/spec of 80% and 82% in diagnosing malignancy in patients with biliary colic or chronic cholecystitis with inconclusive CT or ultrasonography imaging.[46]

Incidental gallbladder cancer is rare, occurring at a rate of 0.7% in cholecystectomies performed for benign disease.[47] When incidental lesions are discovered, reresection is often required. Data from Tata Memorial suggest that PET/CT imaging may be useful in pretreatment evaluation for the extent of residual disease, with a sensitivity of 100% and positive predictive value (PPV) of 91%.[48]

PANCREATIC CANCER
Staging

Primary work-up of a suspected pancreatic neoplasm can include PET/CT imaging, which is used to supplement more well-established imaging modalities such as CT and MR imaging.[49] PET/CT can be particularly useful when differentiating malignant primary tumors from benign entities such as intraductal papillary mucinous neoplasm or pancreatitis. PET/CT has also been shown to detect lesions missed by CT, altering the treatment course of those previously deemed resectable. Retrospective analyses, large meta-analyses, and 1 large prospective trial have shown improved sens/spec of 89% to 91% and 71% to 88% for detection of distant metastases, leading to a change in clinical management in 11% to 50% of cases.[50–57] **Table 2** summarizes the sens/spec of staging PET/CT for pancreatic cancer.

Treatment Planning and Response Evaluation

PET can also be used for radiation treatment planning purposes, particularly when radiotherapy is used in the adjuvant or neoadjuvant settings. PET may be fused with planning CT simulation images for more precise target delineation. A four-dimensional PET scan may also be used to account for tumor motion.[58]

The use of PET to assess treatment response may be useful when attempting to differentiate between residual disease and posttreatment changes. It has been shown in retrospective series that patients with greater PET responses to treatment may have improved survival outcomes,[54,59,60] and these findings have been confirmed in a posthoc analysis of a phase III randomized controlled trial.[61] Other groups have shown that higher baseline SUV values may predict for higher rates of metastatic disease, recurrence, and decreased survival.[56,59,61–67] It has also been shown that high baseline SUV values may predict for improved treatment responses to neoadjuvant and definitive therapies.[53,68,69] The use of PET to assess treatment responses to chemotherapy and/or radiation has been reported in small retrospective series and ranges from 33% to 67%, with a specificity of 84%.[52,58,67]

Posttreatment and Surveillance

Despite the potential advantages of PET in assessing treatment response, it is not routinely recommended.[70] The NCCN guidelines suggest clinical follow-up every 3 to 6 months in the first 2 years after treatment and then every 6 to 12 months thereafter, consisting of a history and physical examination with consideration of monitoring cancer antigen (CA) 19-9 blood marker levels and using CT or MR imaging scanning for surveillance.[49]

However, if clinical recurrence is suspected, PET/CT might be particularly useful when CA 19-9 levels are increasing, especially when CT or MR imaging do not reveal a source of metastatic disease. Several small retrospective studies have shown that PET/CT imaging has superior sensitivity when identifying metastatic lesions compared with CT or MR imaging. In this scenario, PET/CT imaging sens/spec to detect recurrence range from 91% to 98% and 90% to 100%, respectively, which compares favorably with CT sens/spec, which ranges from 55% to 85% and 67% to 85%.[62,71–76]

Colorectal Carcinoma

Staging
In colorectal cancer, the NCCN guidelines state that the use of PET/CT for initial staging is not routinely indicated.[77] PET/CT is given consideration (1) when a patient is unable to receive gadolinium-enhanced MR imaging, (2) to evaluate equivocal CT/MR imaging findings, and (3) in select cases in which there is potentially surgically curable M1 disease.[78] In addition, they do not recommend restaging PET/CT, but offer it as an option in the setting of an increased carcinoembryonic antigen (CEA) level with no evidence of disease recurrence on contrast-enhanced CT, or in cases of distant recurrences amenable to surgical resection. PET/CT for initial staging is most beneficial for clarifying the burden of metastatic disease, especially in patients with hepatic oligometastases amenable to curative-intent surgical resection, stereotactic body radiation therapy, or other aggressive local therapies. In 1 meta-analysis by Niekel and colleagues,[78] sensitivity in detecting liver metastases did not differ by use of CT, MR imaging, and PET/CT on a per-lesion basis, but PET/CT was significantly more sensitive on a per-patient basis (94.2% vs 81.2%). Although individual studies have shown mixed results,[79,80] another meta-analysis of patients with colorectal cancer with hepatic metastasis corroborated the benefit of PET on a per-patient basis (sens/spec of 93% and 86%), with altered management in about 25% of patients.[81] Patel and colleagues[82] reported sens/spec of 75% to 89% and 95%, respectively, for overall staging. Both sens/spec (91%–100% and 75%–100%) were greater for liver metastases. A meta-analysis by Floriani and colleagues[83] showed that PET/CT was superior to ultrasonography, CT, and MR imaging on a per-patient basis for liver metastases, with sens/spec of 95.6% and 98.7%, respectively. A summary of sens/spec from these studies is provided in **Table 2**.

Prognostic response to therapy

Many studies show the ability of PET to identify responders versus nonresponders, both during and following neoadjuvant chemoradiation.[84–86] Limited data suggest that earlier response during neoadjuvant therapy may predict pathologic complete response (pCR).[84,87] One review showed the prognostic value of PET response, which predicted for improved overall and disease-free survival in responders.[85] Although correlation between any metabolic response and pCR has been observed, studies showing this were either small in sample size or did not reach statistical significance.[86,88] Overall, there are insufficient data to recommend PET as a tool for pCR prediction. Future improvements in imaging techniques may allow reliable prognostication of pCR and a change in treatment paradigm.[85]

Posttreatment and surveillance

Although PET/CT is not routinely used for surveillance imaging, it has been extensively studied in the setting of suspected recurrences.[89–91] Multiple studies have proved its usefulness in establishing recurrence in the setting of increased CEA level and negative or equivocal findings on CT or MR imaging.[92–94] In 1 study, 88 patients with increased CEA level and negative or equivocal imaging underwent PET with sens/spec for detection of occult recurrence of 88% and 88%, respectively, with 70% of these patients proceeding to curative-intent salvage therapy. A larger meta-analysis showed sens/spec of 94% and 77% with PET/CT. Different studies have advised different cutoffs for CEA levels. One group specifically determined a level of 3.5 ng/mL to represent the best compromise between sens/spec using receiver operating characteristic curve analysis.[95] Another small but interesting study showed that PET was able to detect local tumor recurrence as well as a 99mTc-labeled CEA antibody fragment, with superior distant metastasis detection.[92] Overall, the use of PET to evaluate recurrence with increased CEA level is well supported, especially when other work-up is equivocal.

Anal Cancer

Staging

PET/CT is superior to conventional imaging studies such as CT for initial staging of anal cancer.[96,97] The primary tumor is often inadequately delineated by CT, especially for large and deeply invasive tumors. In addition, nodal involvement cannot be accurately determined based on size criteria alone using CT, and CT is also more limited in detecting occult distant metastasis in many patients.

Nguyen and colleagues[98] showed that FDG avidity allowed well-delineated primary tumors in 98% of patients with anal cancer, whereas only 58% had clearly determined primary tumors on CT, and these results were corroborated by groups at Washington University (91% and 59%, respectively)[99] and Kaiser Permanente (95% and 64%, respectively).[100] In addition, PET/CT upstaged 17% of patients with pelvic/inguinal nodal disease undetected by CT.[98] Goldman and colleagues[100] found that although 68 patients had FDG-avid locoregional nodes, only 41 of these had enlarged nodes by CT (60.3%). Similarly, Cotter and colleagues[99] reported that PET/CT indicated nodal involvement in about 20% of groins that were normal on CT or physical examination. These results are supported by several recently published systemic reviews and meta-analyses; Mahmud and colleagues[101] reported higher sensitivity (pooled sensitivity 99% for primary, 93% for inguinal nodes) of PET/CT in visualizing the primary tumor and detecting locoregional nodal involvement. Jones and colleagues[102] found that CT and PET/CT had a sensitivity of 60% and 99%, respectively, for detection of the primary tumor, whereas PET/CT led to a change in nodal staging in 28% of patients; PET also identified occult distant metastasis in 3% of patients. The sens/spec findings for all anal cancer studies noted earlier are summarized in **Table 2**.

The European Society for Medical Oncology, European Society of Surgical Oncology, and European Society of Radiotherapy and Oncology (ESMO-ESSO-ESTRO) Clinical Practice Guidelines were updated to include PET as an "optimal but often recommended" tool for initial staging of anal cancer that can alter treatment intent in about 3% to 5% of cases.[103] In addition, the NCCN guidelines recommend that PET/CT be considered for initial staging of anal cancer.[104]

Radiation therapy

PET/CT should be considered for radiation target volume delineation versus CT alone.[39,97,104–107] Krengli and colleagues[108] reported that, among 27 patients with anal cancer, PET/CT resulted in GTV and clinical target volume (CTV) contour changes in 55.6% and 37% of cases, respectively. Furthermore, the GTV and CTV volumes were significantly larger than what was drawn on CT alone ($P = .00006$). Similarly, a study from Royal United Hospital in the United Kingdom found that PET altered the radiation fields in 8 of 61 patients (13%).[109] Investigators from Switzerland found that PET/CT provided information that led to major changes in treatment planning in 17% of patients.[107] A systemic review and meta-analysis

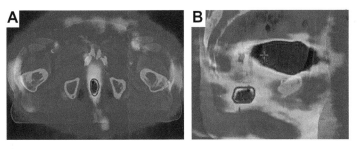

Fig. 2. Staging PET/CT of a patient diagnosed with a localized anal squamous cell carcinoma with the GTV outlined for radiation treatment planning in the axial (*A*) and sagittal planes (*B*).

by Albertsson and colleagues[106] reported that PET/CT changes the target definition in about 1 out of 4 patients, although the investigators did not report data showing how these changes affect OS, tumor control, or quality of life. **Fig. 2** shows GTV delineation with the aid of PET/CT for a patient with localized anal squamous cell carcinoma.

Posttreatment assessment

Although controversial, PET/CT for metabolic response has been reported by several groups to be closely associated with clinical outcomes. Schwarz and colleagues[110] showed that 83% of patients with anal cancer had a complete metabolic response by PET after a mean follow-up of 2.1 months from definitive chemoradiotherapy (CRT) with significantly improved cause-specific survival (CSS) compared with those with an incomplete response (*P*<.01). Nguyen and colleagues[98] found that complete PET response was associated with significantly improved progression-free survival (PFS) compared with patients with partial PET responses. Goldman and colleagues[100] reported that 2-year PFS for patients with complete PET response versus incomplete PET response a mean 12.7 weeks after CRT was 89.8% versus 69.2%, respectively (*P* = .004), whereas 2-year OS was 94.8% versus 79.3% (*P* = .036). A systematic review by Mahmud and colleagues[101] found consistently across all studies that lack of complete PET response in several studies was predictive of PFS, CSS, and OS. However, there is concern that early PET scans could detect residual disease that may resolve without additional treatment over time, leading to unnecessary biopsies or even surgery. Goldman and colleagues[100] showed that the PPV was only 40% for posttreatment PET/CT done within 12 weeks after CRT, whereas it was 52.9% if done 13 to 25 weeks after CRT, suggesting a more prudent approach is to wait for 3 months before using PET/CT to assess for treatment response.

SUMMARY

The role of PET/CT in GI malignancies will continue to evolve as treatment paradigms shift and diagnostic imaging technology improves. More large-scale prospective studies are needed to better define the role of diagnostic PET/CT scanning in the management of GI malignancies, and the authors are optimistic that future studies will help to broaden the impact of PET/CT in the work-up, staging, treatment planning, and monitoring of cancers of the GI tract, particularly as newer metabolic agents (eg, fluorothymidine radiotracers[111]) become available. In the current era, the strongest evidence for PET/CT in GI malignancies is in the staging (especially the diagnosis of metastatic disease, which is occult on other imaging modalities) of esophageal and anal malignancies, treatment planning for anal malignancies, and recurrence monitoring for colorectal and anal malignancies.

REFERENCES

1. Ferlay J, Colombet M, Soerjomataram I, et al. Estimating the global cancer incidence and mortality in 2018: GLOBOCAN sources and methods. Int J Cancer 2019;144(8):1941–53. https://doi.org/10.1002/ijc.31937.
2. Lancet T. Globocan 2018: counting the toll of cancer. Lancet 2018;392(10152):985.
3. Siegel RL, Miller KD, Jemal A. Cancer statistics, 2019. CA Cancer J Clin 2019;69(1):7–34.
4. Phelps ME, Huang SC, Hoffman EJ, et al. Tomographic measurement of local cerebral glucose metabolic rate in humans with (F-18)2-fluoro-2-deoxy-D-glucose: validation of method. Ann Neurol 1979;6(5):371–88.
5. Reivich M, Kuhl D, Wolf A, et al. The [18F]fluorodeoxyglucose method for the measurement of local cerebral glucose utilization in man. Circ Res 1979;44(1):127–37.
6. Townsend DW. Combined positron emission tomography–computed tomography: the historical perspective. Semin Ultrasound CT MR 2008;29(4):232–5.
7. Ajani JA, D'Amico TA, Bentrem DJ, et al. Esophageal and esophagogastric junction cancers, version 2.2019, NCCN clinical practice guidelines in oncology. J Natl Compr Canc Netw 2019;17(7). 855–833.

8. Puli SR, Reddy JBK, Bechtold ML, et al. Staging accuracy of esophageal cancer by endoscopic ultrasound: a meta-analysis and systematic review. World J Gastroenterol 2008;14(10): 1479–90.

9. Van Westreenen HL, Westerterp M, Bossuyt PMM, et al. Systematic review of the staging performance of 18F- fluorodeoxyglucose positron emission tomography in esophageal cancer. J Clin Oncol 2004;22(18):3805–12.

10. Weber WA, Ott K. Imaging of esophageal and gastric cancer. Semin Oncol 2004;31(4):530–41.

11. Lowe VJ, Booya F, Fletcher JG, et al. Comparison of positron emission tomography, computed tomography, and endoscopic ultrasound in the initial staging of patients with esophageal cancer. Mol Imaging Biol 2005;7(6):422–30.

12. Van Vliet EPM, Heijenbrok-Kal MH, Hunink MGM, et al. Staging investigations for oesophageal cancer: a meta-analysis. Br J Cancer 2008;98(3): 547–57.

13. Block MI, Patterson GA, Sundaresan RS, et al. Improvement in staging of esophageal cancer with the addition of positron emission tomography. Ann Thorac Surg 1997;64(3):770–6 [discussion: 776–7].

14. Konski A, Doss M, Milestone B, et al. The integration of 18-fluoro-deoxy-glucose positron emission tomography and endoscopic ultrasound in the treatment-planning process for esophageal carcinoma. Int J Radiat Oncol Biol Phys 2005;61(4): 1123–8.

15. Lordick F, Ott K, Krause B-J, et al. PET to assess early metabolic response and to guide treatment of adenocarcinoma of the oesophagogastric junction: the MUNICON phase II trial. Lancet Oncol 2007;8(9):797–805.

16. Bruzzi JF, Swisher SG, Truong MT, et al. Detection of interval distant metastases: clinical utility of integrated CT-PET imaging in patients with esophageal carcinoma after neoadjuvant therapy. Cancer 2007;109(1):125–34.

17. Kroese TE, Goense L, Van Hillegersberg R, et al. Detection of distant interval metastases after neoadjuvant therapy for esophageal cancer with 18 F-FDG PET(/CT): a systematic review and meta-analysis. Dis Esophagus 2018;31(12).

18. Goense L, van Rossum PSN, Reitsma JB, et al. Diagnostic performance of 18F-FDG PET and PET/CT for the detection of recurrent esophageal cancer after treatment with curative intent: a systematic review and meta-analysis. J Nucl Med 2015;56(7):995–1002.

19. National Comprehensive Cancer Network. Gastric Cancer (Version 2.2019). Available at: http://www.nccn.org/professionals/physician_gls/pdf/gastric.pdf. Accessed June 01, 2019.

20. Dassen AE, Lips DJ, Hoekstra CJ, et al. FDG-PET has no definite role in preoperative imaging in gastric cancer. Eur J Surg Oncol 2009;35(5):449–55.

21. Altini C, Asabella AN, Di Palo A, et al. 18F-FDG PET/CT role in staging of gastric carcinomas: comparison with conventional contrast enhancement computed tomography. Medicine (Baltimore) 2015;94(20):e864.

22. Wu C-X, Zhu Z-H. Diagnosis and evaluation of gastric cancer by positron emission tomography. World J Gastroenterol 2014;20(16):4574.

23. Yun M. Imaging of gastric cancer metabolism using 18 F-FDG PET/CT. J Gastric Cancer 2014; 14(1):1.

24. Hocazade C, Özdemir N, Yazici O, et al. Concordance of positron emission tomography and computed tomography in patients with locally advanced gastric and esophageal cancer. Ann Nucl Med 2015;29(7):621–6.

25. Chen J, Cheong J-H, Yun MJ, et al. Improvement in preoperative staging of gastric adenocarcinoma with positron emission tomography. Cancer 2005; 103(11):2383–90.

26. Hopkins S, Yang GY. FDG PET imaging in the staging and management of gastric cancer. J Gastrointest Oncol 2011;2(1):39–44.

27. Kinkel K, Lu Y, Both M, et al. Detection of hepatic metastases from cancers of the gastrointestinal tract by using noninvasive imaging methods (US, CT, MR Imaging, PET): a meta-analysis. Radiology 2002;224(3):748–56.

28. Findlay JM, Antonowicz S, Segaran A, et al. Routinely staging gastric cancer with 18F-FDG PET-CT detects additional metastases and predicts early recurrence and death after surgery. Eur Radiol 2019;29(5):2490–8.

29. Ott K, Herrmann K, Lordick F, et al. Early metabolic response evaluation by Fluorine-18 fluorodeoxyglucose positron emission tomography allows in vivo testing of chemosensitivity in gastric cancer: long-term results of a prospective study. Clin Cancer Res 2008;14(7):2012–8.

30. Won E, Shah MA, Schöder H, et al. Use of positron emission tomography scan response to guide treatment change for locally advanced gastric cancer: the Memorial Sloan Kettering Cancer Center experience. J Gastrointest Oncol 2016;7(4): 506–14.

31. De Potter T, Flamen P, Van Cutsem E, et al. Whole-body PET with FDG for the diagnosis of recurrent gastric cancer. Eur J Nucl Med Mol Imaging 2002;29(4):525–9.

32. Sim SH, Kim YJ, Oh D-Y, et al. The role of PET/CT in detection of gastric cancer recurrence. BMC Cancer 2009;9:73.

33. Smyth EC, Verheij M, Allum W, et al. Gastric cancer: ESMO clinical practice guidelines for

diagnosis, treatment and follow-up†. Ann Oncol 2016;27(suppl_5):v38–49.

34. Allum WH, Blazeby JM, Griffin SM, et al. Guidelines for the management of oesophageal and gastric cancer. Gut 2011;60(11):1449–72.

35. Baiocchi GL, Marrelli D, Verlato G, et al. Follow-up after gastrectomy for cancer: an appraisal of the Italian research group for gastric cancer. Ann Surg Oncol 2014;21(6):2005–11.

36. Donswijk ML, Hess S, Mulders T, et al. [1 8 F]Fluorodeoxyglucose PET/computed tomography in gastrointestinal malignancies. PET Clin 2014;9(4): 421–41.

37. Nishiyama Y, Yamamoto Y, Kimura N, et al. Comparison of early and delayed FDG PET for evaluation of biliary stricture. Nucl Med Commun 2007; 28(12):914–9.

38. Moon CM, Bang S, Chung JB, et al. Usefulness of 18 F-fluorodeoxyglucose positron emission tomography in differential diagnosis and staging of cholangiocarcinomas. J Gastroenterol Hepatol 2008; 23(5):759–65.

39. Lambrecht M, Haustermans K. Clinical evidence on PET-CT for radiation therapy planning in gastro-intestinal tumors. Radiother Oncol 2010; 96(3):339–46.

40. Onal C, Topuk S, Yapar AF, et al. Comparison of computed tomography- and positron emission tomography-based radiotherapy planning in cholangiocarcinoma. Onkologie 2013;36(9):484–90.

41. Khan MA, Combs CS, Brunt EM, et al. Positron emission tomography scanning in the evaluation of hepatocellular carcinoma. J Hepatol 2000;32(5):792–7.

42. Izuishi K, Yamamoto Y, Mori H, et al. Molecular mechanisms of [18F]fluorodeoxyglucose accumulation in liver cancer. Oncol Rep 2014;31(2):701–6.

43. Kim JY, Kim M-H, Lee TY, et al. Clinical role of 18 F-FDG PET-CT in suspected and potentially operable cholangiocarcinoma: a prospective study compared with conventional imaging. Am J Gastroenterol 2008;103:1145–51.

44. Corvera CU, Blumgart LH, Akhurst T, et al. 18F-fluorodeoxyglucose positron emission tomography influences management decisions in patients with biliary cancer. J Am Coll Surg 2008;206(1):57–65.

45. Song J-Y, Lee YN, Kim YS, et al. Predictability of preoperative 18F-FDG PET for histopathological differentiation and early recurrence of primary malignant intrahepatic tumors. Nucl Med Commun 2015;36(4):319–27.

46. Rodríguez-Fernández A, Gómez-Río M, Llamas-Elvira M, et al. Positron-emission tomography with fluorine-18-fluoro-2-deoxy-D-glucose for gallbladder cancer diagnosis. Am J Surg 2004;188(2): 171–5.

47. Choi KS, Choi SB, Park P, et al. Clinical characteristics of incidental or unsuspected gallbladder cancers diagnosed during or after cholecystectomy: a systematic review and meta-analysis. World J Gastroenterol 2015;21(4):1315–23.

48. Shukla PJ, Barreto SG, Arya S, et al. Does PET-CT scan have a role prior to radical re-resection for incidental gallbladder cancer? HPB (Oxford) 2008;10(6):439–45.

49. National Comprehensive Cancer Network. Pancreatic Cancer (Version 2.2019). Available at: http://www.nccn.org/professionals/physician_gls/ pdf/pancreatic.pdf. Accessed June 01, 2019.

50. Gambhir SS, Czernin J, Schwimmer J, et al. A tabulated summary of the FDG PET literature. J Nucl Med 2001;42(5 Suppl):1S–93S.

51. Tang S, Huang G, Liu J, et al. Usefulness of 18F-FDG PET, combined FDG-PET/CT and EUS in diagnosing primary pancreatic carcinoma: a meta-analysis. Eur J Radiol 2011;78(1):142–50.

52. Farma JM, Santillan AA, Melis M, et al. PET/CT fusion scan enhances CT staging in patients with pancreatic neoplasms. Ann Surg Oncol 2008;15(9):2465–71.

53. Kurahara H, Maemura K, Mataki Y, et al. Significance of 18F-Fluorodeoxyglucose (FDG) uptake in response to chemoradiotherapy for pancreatic cancer. Ann Surg Oncol 2019;26(2):644–51.

54. Bang S, Chung HW, Park SW, et al. The clinical usefulness of 18-Fluorodeoxyglucose positron emission tomography in the differential diagnosis, staging, and response evaluation after concurrent chemoradiotherapy for pancreatic cancer. J Clin Gastroenterol 2006;40(10):923–9.

55. Ghaneh P, Hanson R, Titman A, et al. PET-PANC: multicentre prospective diagnostic accuracy and health economic analysis study of the impact of combined modality 18fluorine-2-fluoro-2-deoxy-d-glucose positron emission tomography with computed tomography scanning in the diagnosis and management of pancreatic cancer. Health Technol Assess (Rockv) 2018;22(7):1–114.

56. Kim HR, Seo M, Nah YW, et al. Clinical impact of fluorine-18-fluorodeoxyglucose positron emission tomography/computed tomography in patients with resectable pancreatic cancer. Nucl Med Commun 2018;39(7):691–8.

57. Wang L, Dong P, Wang WG, et al. Positron emission tomography modalities prevent futile radical resection of pancreatic cancer: a meta-analysis. Int J Surg 2017;46:119–25.

58. Kishi T, Matsuo Y, Nakamura A, et al. Comparative evaluation of respiratory-gated and ungated FDG-PET for target volume definition in radiotherapy treatment planning for pancreatic cancer. Radiother Oncol 2016;120(2):217–21.

59. Maemura K, Takao S, Shinchi H, et al. Role of positron emission tomography in decisions on treatment strategies for pancreatic cancer. J Hepatobiliary Pancreat Surg 2006;13(5):435–41.

60. Topkan E, Parlak C, Kotek A, et al. Predictive value of metabolic 18FDG-PET response on outcomes in patients with locally advanced pancreatic carcinoma treated with definitive concurrent chemoradiotherapy. BMC Gastroenterol 2011;11(1):123.

61. Ramanathan RK, Goldstein D, Korn RL, et al. Positron emission tomography response evaluation from a randomized phase III trial of weekly nab-paclitaxel plus gemcitabine versus gemcitabine alone for patients with metastatic adenocarcinoma of the pancreas. Ann Oncol 2016;27(4): 648–53.

62. Sperti C, Pasquali C, Bissoli S, et al. Tumor relapse after pancreatic cancer resection is detected earlier by 18-FDG PET than by CT. J Gastrointest Surg 2010;14(1):131–40.

63. Wang Z, Chen J-Q, Liu J-L, et al. FDG-PET in diagnosis, staging and prognosis of pancreatic carcinoma: a meta-analysis. World J Gastroenterol 2013;19(29):4808.

64. Ariake K, Motoi F, Shimomura H, et al. 18-Fluorodeoxyglucose positron emission tomography predicts recurrence in resected pancreatic ductal adenocarcinoma. J Gastrointest Surg 2018;22(2):279–87.

65. Omiya Y, Ichikawa S, Satoh Y, et al. Prognostic value of preoperative fluorodeoxyglucose positron emission tomography/computed tomography in patients with potentially resectable pancreatic cancer. Abdom Radiol (NY) 2018;43(12):3381–9.

66. Albano D, Familiari D, Gentile R, et al. Clinical and prognostic value of 18F-FDG-PET/CT in restaging of pancreatic cancer. Nucl Med Commun 2018; 39(8):741–6.

67. Chirindel A, Alluri KC, Chaudhry MA, et al. Prognostic value of FDG PET/CT–derived parameters in pancreatic adenocarcinoma at initial PET/CT staging. Am J Roentgenol 2015;204(5):1093–9.

68. Heinrich S, Goerres GW, Schäfer M, et al. Positron emission tomography/computed tomography influences on the management of resectable pancreatic cancer and its cost-effectiveness. Ann Surg 2005;242(2):235–43.

69. Kittaka H, Takahashi H, Ohigashi H, et al. Role of 18F-Fluorodeoxyglucose positron emission tomography/computed tomography in predicting the pathologic response to preoperative chemoradiation therapy in patients with resectable T3 pancreatic cancer. World J Surg 2013;37(1): 169–78.

70. Rijkers AP, Valkema R, Duivenvoorden HJ, et al. Usefulness of F-18-fluorodeoxyglucose positron emission tomography to confirm suspected pancreatic cancer: a meta-analysis. Eur J Surg Oncol 2014;40(7):794–804.

71. Asagi A, Ohta K, Nasu J, et al. Utility of contrast-enhanced FDG-PET/CT in the clinical management of pancreatic cancer. Pancreas 2013;42(1):11–9.

72. Jadvar H, Fischman AJ. Evaluation of pancreatic carcinoma with FDG PET. Abdom Imaging 2001; 26(3):254–9.

73. Ruf J, Hänninen EL, Oettle H, et al. Detection of recurrent pancreatic cancer: comparison of FDG-PET with CT/MRI. Pancreatology 2005;5(2–3):266–72.

74. Kitajima K, Murakami K, Yamasaki E, et al. Performance of integrated FDG-PET/contrast-enhanced CT in the diagnosis of recurrent pancreatic cancer: comparison with integrated FDG-PET/non-contrast-enhanced CT and enhanced CT. Mol Imaging Biol 2010;12(4):452–9.

75. Rayamajhi S, Balachandran A, Katz M, et al. Utility of (18) F-FDG PET/CT and CECT in conjunction with serum CA 19-9 for detecting recurrent pancreatic adenocarcinoma. Abdom Radiol (NY) 2018; 43(2):505–13.

76. Jung W, Jang J-Y, Kang MJ, et al. The clinical usefulness of 18F-fluorodeoxyglucose positron emission tomography-computed tomography (PET-CT) in follow-up of curatively resected pancreatic cancer patients. HPB (Oxford) 2016;18(1):57–64.

77. National Comprehensive Cancer Network. Colon Cancer (Version 2.2019). Available at: http://www.nccn.org/professionals/physician_gls/pdf/colon.pdf. Accessed June 01, 2019.

78. Niekel MC, Bipat S, Stoker J. Diagnostic imaging of colorectal liver metastases with CT, MR imaging, FDG PET, and/or FDG PET/CT: a meta-analysis of prospective studies including patients who have not previously undergone treatment. Radiology 2010;257(3):674–84.

79. Moulton CA, Gu CS, Law CH, et al. Effect of PET before liver resection on surgical management for colorectal adenocarcinoma metastases a randomized clinical trial. JAMA 2014;311(18):1863–9.

80. Joyce DL, Wahl RL, Patel PV, et al. Preoperative positron emission tomography to evaluate potentially resectable hepatic colorectal metastases. Arch Surg 2006;141(12):1220–6.

81. Maffione AM, Lopci E, Bluemel C, et al. Diagnostic accuracy and impact on management of 18F-FDG PET and PET/CT in colorectal liver metastasis: a meta-analysis and systematic review. Eur J Nucl Med Mol Imaging 2015;42(1):152–63.

82. Patel S, McCall M, Ohinmaa A, et al. Positron emission tomography/computed tomographic scans compared to computed tomographic scans for detecting colorectal liver metastases. Ann Surg 2011; 253(4):666–71.

83. Floriani I, Torri V, Rulli E, et al. Performance of imaging modalities in diagnosis of liver metastases from colorectal cancer: a systematic review and meta-analysis. J Magn Reson Imaging 2010;31(1): 19–31.

84. Joye I, Deroose CM, Vandecaveye V, et al. The role of diffusion-weighted MRI and 18F-FDG PET/CT in

the prediction of pathologic complete response after radiochemotherapy for rectal cancer: a systematic review. Radiother Oncol 2014;113(2):158–65.

85. Memon S, Lynch AC, Akhurst T, et al. Systematic review of FDG-PET prediction of complete pathological response and survival in rectal cancer. Ann Surg Oncol 2014;21(11):3598–607.

86. Mak D, Joon DL, Chao M, et al. The use of PET in assessing tumor response after neoadjuvant chemoradiation for rectal cancer. Radiother Oncol 2010;97(2):205–11.

87. Hatt M, Van Stiphout R, Le Pogam A, et al. Early prediction of pathological response in locally advanced rectal cancer based on sequential 18F-FDG PET. Acta Oncol (Madr) 2013;52(3):619–26.

88. Konski A, Li T, Sigurdson E, et al. Use of molecular imaging to predict clinical outcome in patients with rectal cancer after preoperative chemotherapy and radiation. Int J Radiat Oncol Biol Phys 2009;74(1): 55–9.

89. Patel K, Hadar N, Lee J, et al. The lack of evidence for PET or PET/CT surveillance of patients with treated lymphoma, colorectal cancer, and head and neck cancer: a systematic review. J Nucl Med 2013;54(9):1518–27.

90. Pfister DG, Benson AB, Somerfield MR. Surveillance strategies after curative treatment of colorectal cancer. N Engl J Med 2004;350(23):2375–82.

91. Pelosi E, Deandreis D. The role of 18F-fluoro-deoxy-glucose positron emission tomography (FDG-PET) in the management of patients with colorectal cancer. Eur J Surg Oncol 2007;33(1):1–6.

92. Willkomm P, Bender H, Bangard M, et al. FDG PET and immunoscintigraphy with 99mTc-labeled antibody fragments for detection of the recurrence of colorectal carcinoma. J Nucl Med 2000;41(10): 1657–63.

93. Lu YY, Chen JH, Chien CR, et al. Use of FDG-PET or PET/CT to detect recurrent colorectal cancer in patients with elevated CEA: a systematic review and meta-analysis. Int J Colorectal Dis 2013; 28(8):1039–47.

94. Khan K, Athauda A, Aitken K. Survival outcomes in asymptomatic patients with normal conventional imaging but raised carcinoembryonic antigen levels in colorectal cancer following positron emission tomography-computed tomography imaging. Oncologist 2016;21(12):1502–8.

95. Chiaravalloti A, Fiorentini A, Palombo E, et al. Evaluation of recurrent disease in the re-staging of colorectal cancer by 18F-FDG PET/CT: use of CEA and CA 19-9 in patient selection. Oncol Lett 2016;12(5):4209–13.

96. Trautmann TG, Zuger JH. Positron emission tomography for pretreatment staging and posttreatment evaluation in cancer of the anal canal. Mol Imaging Biol 2005;7(4):309–13.

97. Grigsby PW. FDG-PET/CT: new horizons in anal cancer. Gastroenterol Clin Biol 2009;33(5):456–8.

98. Nguyen BT, Joon DL, Khoo V, et al. Assessing the impact of FDG-PET in the management of anal cancer. Radiother Oncol 2008;87(3):376–82.

99. Cotter SE, Grigsby PW, Siegel BA, et al. FDG-PET/CT in the evaluation of anal carcinoma. Int J Radiat Oncol 2006;65(3):720–5.

100. Goldman KE, White EC, Rao AR, et al. Posttreatment FDG-PET-CT response is predictive of tumor progression and survival in anal carcinoma. Pract Radiat Oncol 2016;6(5):e149–54.

101. Mahmud A, Poon R, Jonker D. PET imaging in anal canal cancer: a systematic review and meta-analysis. Br J Radiol 2017;90(1080):20170370.

102. Jones M, Hruby G, Solomon M, et al. The role of FDG-PET in the initial staging and response assessment of anal cancer: a systematic review and meta-analysis. Ann Surg Oncol 2015;22(11): 3574–81.

103. Glynne-Jones R, Nilsson PJ, Aschele C, et al. Anal cancer: ESMO–ESSO–ESTRO clinical practice guidelines for diagnosis, treatment and follow-up. Radiother Oncol 2014;111(3):330–9.

104. Benson AB, Venook AP, Al-Hawary MM, et al. Anal carcinoma, Version 2.2018, NCCN clinical practice guidelines in oncology. J Natl Compr Canc Netw 2018;16(7):852–71.

105. Speirs CK, Grigsby PW, Huang J, et al. PET-based radiation therapy planning. PET Clin 2015;10(1): 27–44.

106. Albertsson P, Alverbratt C, Liljegren A, et al. Positron emission tomography and computed tomographic (PET/CT) imaging for radiation therapy planning in anal cancer: a systematic review and meta-analysis. Crit Rev Oncol Hematol 2018;126: 6–12.

107. Zimmermann M, Beer J, Bodis S, et al. PET-CT guided SIB-IMRT combined with concurrent 5-FU/MMC for the treatment of anal cancer. Acta Oncol (Madr) 2017;56(12):1734–40.

108. Krengli M, Milia ME, Turri L, et al. FDG-PET/CT imaging for staging and target volume delineation in conformal radiotherapy of anal carcinoma. Radiat Oncol 2010;5(1):10.

109. Winton E de, Heriot AG, Ng M, et al. The impact of 18-fluorodeoxyglucose positron emission tomography on the staging, management and outcome of anal cancer. Br J Cancer 2009;100(5):693–700.

110. Schwarz JK, Siegel BA, Dehdashti F, et al. Tumor response and survival predicted by post-therapy FDG-PET/CT in anal cancer. Int J Radiat Oncol 2008;71(1):180–6.

111. Herrmann K, Ott K, Buck AK, et al. Imaging gastric cancer with PET and the radiotracers 18F-FLT and 18F-FDG: a comparative analysis. J Nucl Med 2007;48(12):1945–50.

Evolving Role of Novel Quantitative PET Techniques to Detect Radiation-Induced Complications

Alexandra D. Dreyfuss, BS[a,1], Pegah Jahangiri, MD[a,1], Charles B. Simone II, MD[b,*], Abass Alavi, MD[a]

KEYWORDS

- Radiation therapy • Complications • Radiation-induced lung injury • Cardiovascular • PET/CT
- Radiation oncology

KEY POINTS

- PET-based novel quantitative techniques can be used to detect radiation-induced complications.
- PET has an increasingly recognized but integral role in assessing the lung inflammatory changes induced by radiation therapy, which manifest as increased ^{18}F-fluorodeoxyglucose uptake in lung parenchyma.
- PET also has an emerging role in the detection of radiation-induced cardiovascular toxicity.

INTRODUCTION

Radiation therapy (RT) has proved to be highly effective in treating a variety of malignancies either alone or in combination with surgery and/or systemic therapy. Radiation causes DNA damage by increasing oxidative stress and free radical formation, inducing cell death through an interplay between apoptosis, necrosis, autophagy, and senescence.[1,2] This process is followed by a cascade of inflammatory events, including tissue infiltration by neutrophils and macrophages, and the associated release of cytokines (interleukin [IL]-1, IL-6, tumor necrosis factor alpha [TNF-α]).[3–8] Therefore, RT tolerability is contingent on the selective targeting of tumor cells and the sparing of surrounding normal tissue. However, dose delivery to nearby structures is often unavoidable, even with the development of more advanced RT technologies, including intensity-modulated RT (IMRT), stereotactic body radiation therapy (SBRT), and proton therapy. The resulting normal tissue damage from this incidental irradiation contributes to significant toxicities and decreases in quality of life in many patients.

Radiation-induced normal tissue toxicities can vary greatly in terms of pathophysiologic determinants and timing of disease development, both of which are influenced by the radiation dose and volume of normal tissues receiving irradiation and largely depend on the baseline rate of turnover of the tissues involved. For example, in the highly proliferative gastrointestinal tract, high-grade radiotherapy-induced toxicities often manifest acutely and subacutely as ulcers, hemorrhages, or perforations, because high-turnover mucosal

Disclosure: The authors have nothing to disclose.
[a] Department of Radiology, Hospital of the University of Pennsylvania, University of Pennsylvania, 3400 Spruce Street, Philadelphia, PA 19104, USA; [b] Department of Radiation Oncology, New York Proton Center, 225 East 126th Street, New York, NY 10035, USA
[1] These authors contributed equally as cofirst authors.
* Corresponding author.
E-mail address: csimone@nyproton.com

cells are rapidly eliminated.[9] This area is in contrast with the pulmonary and cardiovascular systems, whose susceptibility to radiation injury is often a major constraining factor in treatment planning. Radiation-induced lung injury is dose limiting for the treatment of lung cancer and other thoracic malignancies and can lead to potentially fatal pneumonitis and quality-of-life-limiting fibrosis. In addition, there is increasing recognition that radiation-induced cardiac injury can lead to quality-of-life-limiting cardiac disease and death from major cardiac events. At present, there are no comprehensive and up-to-date reviews addressing how PET may be used to detect radiation-induced complications. This article focuses on pulmonary and cardiovascular complications of RT and discusses how PET-based novel quantitative techniques can be used to detect these events earlier than current imaging modalities or clinical presentation allow.

PULMONARY COMPLICATIONS OF RADIATION THERAPY

Radiation-induced lung injury (RILI), which includes radiation pneumonitis (RP) and radiation fibrosis, was first described about 120 years ago, shortly after the development of roentgenograms.[10,11] These injuries are observed in patients who have undergone thoracic irradiation for the treatment of lung, breast, esophageal, and other thoracic malignancies, as well as lymphomas. Radiation-induced damage to normal lung parenchyma remains the dose-limiting factor in thoracic radiotherapy and can involve other critical structures within the thorax in addition to the lungs, such as heart, pericardium, large vessels, and esophagus.

A large number of studies describe the histopathologic, biochemical, kinetic, physiologic, and molecular responses of lung cells to ionizing radiation.[12–16] However, the clinical diagnosis of RILI is often complicated by the presence of other conditions, including malignancy, infection, and cardiogenic pulmonary edema.[17] The incidence of RILI varies depending on the particular radiotherapy regimen used and volume of normal lung irradiated. Furthermore, there is a discrepancy between the frequency of clinical pneumonitis and radiographic evidence of RT-induced lung injury. This article focuses on the role of PET-based techniques to detect RILI.

RILI results from the combination of direct toxicity on normal lung tissues and, perhaps more importantly, the development of fibrosis triggered by radiation-induced cellular signal transduction. The cytotoxic effect is largely a consequence of DNA damage that causes death in normal lung epithelial cells. Several different cytokines, such as transforming growth factor beta 1,[18–20] proinflammatory cytokines, TNF-α, IL-1a,[21,22] platelet-derived growth factor, basic fibroblast growth factor,[23,24] interferon-gamma,[25] and cluster of differentiation 40[26] can mediate the formation of fibrosis, which results in the late morbidity of compromising lung function.

The pathologic and clinical changes in the lung following radiation exposure may be divided into the 5 phases: immediate, latent, acute exudative, intermediate, and fibrotic phases. During the first 2 phases, thick secretions accumulate because of an increase in the number of goblet cells combined with ciliary dysfunction within hours to days.[14] The third phase (acute exudative phase) is clinically referred to as RP, which occurs immediately following 6 months or more after radiation exposure and consists of sloughing of endothelial and epithelial cells, narrowing of the pulmonary capillaries, and microvascular thrombosis.[27] In the fourth phase, or intermediate phase, thickening of the interstitium may result, and fibroblasts proliferate within the alveolar walls and spaces.[28,29] A final phase consists of fibrosis that may be evident as early as 6 months following radiation exposure but that can progress over years. The anatomic narrowing of alveolar spaces results in diminishing lung volume, collagen deposition can lead to ventilation-perfusion mismatch and result in worsening of pulmonary function, and vascular subintimal fibrosis and distortion cause capillary dysfunction.[30] Also, organizing pneumonia even in areas outside the radiation port, including the contralateral lung, has been reported approximately 3 to 17 months after irradiation.[31–34]

Although acute and subacute RP usually develops in the weeks to first 6 months following radiation exposure, clinical symptoms of radiation fibrosis develop after 6 to 12 months. The symptoms and signs of the 2 phases are similar and include nonproductive cough, dyspnea, fever, chest pain, malaise, weight loss, crackles, pleural rub, dullness to percussion, tachypnea, cyanosis, and signs of pulmonary hypertension. However, fever is less likely to occur in the fibrotic phase.[35,36]

Method of irradiation, volume of lung irradiated, dose and dose per fraction of irradiation, time-dose factor, and induction and conduction chemotherapy are all factors that may modulate the frequency or severity of RILI following RT. Also, prior thoracic irradiation, volume loss caused by lung collapse, tumor location, younger age, smoking history, poor pretreatment performance status, poor pretreatment lung function, chronic obstructive pulmonary disease (COPD), interstitial lung disease, female sex, endocrine therapy for breast cancer, and glucocorticoid withdrawal during radiotherapy have all been reported to influence the risk of RP.[37,38] An analysis of 318 patients undergoing concurrent chemoradiotherapy showed that 47 patients developed RP but, among those 47, 13 (28%) were confounded by COPD, tumor regrowth/progression, or cardiac disease.[17] Yirmibesoglu and colleagues[39] also evaluated 434 patients with non–small cell lung cancer (NSCLC) receiving thoracic RT and found that 21 (17%) developed clinical RP, but 10 of those (48%) had confounders, including COPD exacerbation, other infection, and tumor progression.

From the factors mentioned earlier, methods of irradiation could be a promising area of further research. Radiation oncologists continue to work to improve the targeting of radiation, increasing the dose given to diseased tissue while sparing normal tissue through the use of advanced treatment modalities and through the optimization of immobilization, margins, and imaging.[40,41]

This general approach of distribution of therapeutic radiation dose within the patient to match the intended target volume as closely as possible while minimizing the dose to other tissues is often referred to as conformal RT (CRT). Clinically significant RP has developed less commonly with more specialized techniques, including IMRT,[42] SBRT,[43] compared with three-dimensional conformal photon RT.[44–48] Also, the use of protons may further decrease the incidence of RP because protons limit tissue penetration and allow more precise dosing.[49–51]

Role of PET in Assessing Radiation-Induced Pulmonary Toxicity

PET has become integrated into multiple aspects of oncology over the last decade. PET imaging has repeatedly been shown to provide improved sensitivity and specificity in diagnosing, staging, RT tumor volume delineation, risk stratification, prognostication, and response monitoring for thoracic malignancies.[52,53] Moreover, it has an emerging but integral role in assessing the extent of inflammatory changes induced by thoracic RT, which manifest as increased ^{18}F-fluorodeoxyglucose (FDG) uptake in lung parenchyma and, thus, is detectable by FDG-PET/computed tomography (CT). Therefore, PET may serve as a predictive tool to identify patients at highest risk of developing RP.[54–59]

As advanced techniques such as IMRT and proton therapy have increased in use, PET/CT scans have played increasingly critical roles in radiation

oncology, particularly in the target delineation of tumors for radiation oncologists delivering therapeutic doses to cancerous cells while minimizing the radiation dose to nearby organs.[60–62] Proton therapy may allow less radiation-induced inflammation and toxicity of adjacent organs at risk compared with other radiotherapy modalities by reducing the doses to normal structures.[49,63]

In recent years some studies have shown the important role of FDG-PET/CT in assessing radiation-induced lung inflammation.[49,54–56,58,59,63–70] Our group, in a pilot study of 20 patients, recently showed that quantification of the global lung parenchymal FDG uptake after photon or proton RT for patients with locally advanced NSCLC can be achieved by subtracting the tumor uptake from the total lung FDG uptake via volume-based quantitative FDG-PET/CT parameters. The results showed statistically significant increases in global lung uptake parameters such as global lung glycolysis, total lesion glycolysis, and lung parenchyma mean standardized uptake value (SUV_{mean}) in the involved irradiated lung but no significant changes in the contralateral, unirradiated lung. Because significant increases in global lung uptake parameters can be identified in the irradiated lung, volumetric PET parameters may be able to serve as potential biomarkers for assessing lung inflammation after RT.[64]

Mac Manus and colleagues[66] used a visual scale of 0 to 3 to correspond with the severity of RP (40% increase in risk of RP for each increase on the 0–3 scale) on post–thoracic RT FDG-PET/CT scans. Their results showed there is significant correlation between intensity of FDG uptake in pulmonary tissue after RT with the presence and severity of RP. Another study of 73 patients with NSCLC who underwent RT showed that increased FDG uptake in normal lung parenchyma (radiosensitivity) was associated with tumor response to RT (radioresponsiveness) on both PET ($P = .0044$) and CT imaging ($P = .029$), suggesting a positive relationship between tumor radioresponsiveness and normal tissue radiosensitivity.[58] In a prospective pilot study, De Ruysscher and colleagues[65] assessed FDG-PET/CT scans, which were taken on days 0, 7, and 14 after initiation of RT in 18 patients with stage III NSCLC. They found that pre-RT SUX_{max} in the lung was not significantly different between patients who developed clinical RILI (6 out of 18) and those who did not. However, those who developed clinical RILI had a significantly increased SUV on days 7 and 14, whereas the other individuals with no development of RILI showed no similar SUV increases.

Guerrero and colleagues,[55] in a detailed study of 36 patients with esophageal cancer undergoing thoracic RT and restaging FDG-PET/CT after 4 to 12 weeks, reported that there was a linear relationship between the uptake of FDG in irradiated lung and the local delivered dose to a prespecified voxel of the lung after chemoradiotherapy (chemoRT). This apparent dose-response relationship supports the use of FDG-PET as a marker for monitoring RP response. Echeverria and colleagues[54] used the same method to identify a positive correlation between clinically apparent proton RT-induced RP in patients with esophageal cancer and pulmonary metabolic radiation response (PMRR). Likewise, McCurdy and colleagues[67] represented a linear relationship of the metabolic RP dose-response from posttreatment FDG-PET/CT imaging of 24 patients with lung cancer.

In a retrospective study of 101 patients with esophageal cancer undergoing restaging FDG-PET/CT 3 to 12 weeks after RT, Hart and colleagues[56] examined the relationship between FDG uptake on post-RT PET imaging, pre-RT radiation dosimetry as assessed using dose-volume histograms, and the subsequent development of clinically symptomatic pneumonitis. Predictably, the investigators found a significant association between increases in the mean lung radiation dose and FDG uptake and RP ($P = .032$ for mean lung radiation dose, $P = .033$ for FDG uptake, respectively); they also found that PMRR was also associated with an increased pneumonitis risk.

The advent of proton therapy, which achieves improvements in localization of radiation dose and reductions in delivered dose to normal tissues, may allow fewer treatment toxicities, specifically RILI, and an increase in effectiveness of treatment compared with photon therapy (**Fig. 1**). Our group recently assessed the feasibility of FDG-PET/CT to quantify radiation-induced pneumonitis in ipsilateral and contralateral lungs of patients with locally advanced NSCLC who received proton or photon RT and showed that proton RT induces less inflammatory response in both the ipsilateral and contralateral lungs of patients compared with photon RT.[49] Another study by Rice and colleagues[63] showed that patients with NSCLC receiving photon RT had significantly increased FDG uptake in their ipsilateral and contralateral lungs, whereas proton RT did not lead to similar increases, suggesting the feasibility of detecting inflammatory responses by PET/CT analysis.

CARDIOVASCULAR COMPLICATIONS OF RADIATION THERAPY

Cardiovascular disease is now reported as the most common nonmalignant cause of death among cancer survivors.[1] For thoracic RT patients in particular, cardiovascular sequelae remain a significant cause of morbidity and mortality.[5,71–75] A recent case-control study assessing 2168 women with breast cancer showed a 7.4% increase in major coronary events with each 1-Gy increase in mean heart radiation dose.[72] In locally advanced NSCLC, decreased survival at 18 months (53.9% vs 66.9%, $P = .007$) with higher radiation doses (74 Gy vs 60 Gy) was postulated to be a function, at least in part, of increased cardiovascular morbidity and mortality.[76] Moreover, in mediastinal lymphoma, patients who received chest RT as part of their treatment had a 4.7 to 19.3 per 10,000 person-years absolute excess risk for undergoing a cardiac procedure.[77]

Cardiovascular manifestations of radiation-induced toxicity are heterogeneous and can present clinically as cardiomyopathies, accelerated coronary artery disease, valvular dysfunction, myocarditis or pericarditis, and conduction system abnormalities, and they can occur anywhere from midtreatment (eg, pericarditis, which sometimes requires treatment breaks or dose reductions) to 20 years or more after RT,[78] with increasing recognition that major cardiac events and death from radiation-induced cardiac disease can happen just months to a year or two after thoracic radiotherapy.[79]

At present, the cardiovascular care of at-risk RT patients is limited and, when performed, is centered around serial measurements of left ventricular ejection fraction with echocardiography along with risk stratification by general cardiovascular risk factors and/or receipt of cardiotoxic medical therapies. However, a glaring deficiency in evidence-based data for clinical decision making and surveillance remains, and early radiomic identification of oncology radiotherapy patients at increased risk of cardiac complications is a pressing clinical challenge.

^{18}F-Fluorodeoxyglucose PET in Radiation-Induced Cardiovascular Disease

An attractive radiomic approach to diagnosing RT-induced cardiovascular toxicity is to implement FDG-PET/CT. For years, FDG-PET has been a focal point for molecular imaging in a wide variety of disease processes, and its capacity to diagnose myocardial inflammation, myocardial perfusion defects, vascular damage, and atherosclerosis (all thought to be fundamental mechanisms in the development of radiation-induced heart disease) makes it uniquely poised to enhance cardio-oncologic care. This article discusses the most prominent studies that show how FDG-PET

A Before and after photon radiotherapy

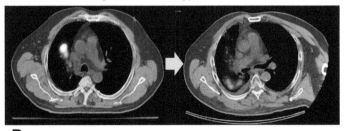

B Before and after proton radiotherapy

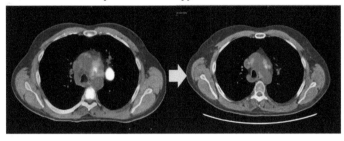

Fig. 1. Radiation-induced lung inflammation (radiation pneumonitis) in 2 patients with non–small cell lung carcinoma. (A) There is obvious lung parenchymal inflammation in the right lung after photon radiotherapy shown on the fused FDG-PET/CT scan. (B) There is no significant lung parenchymal inflammation in left lung after proton radiotherapy on the fused FDG-PET/CT scan.

imaging can be used in the cardiovascular care of radiotherapy oncology patients. A summary of PET studies assessing the cardiovascular complications of RT can be found in **Table 1**.

Myocardial injury: inflammation and ischemic cardiomyopathies

Recently, a significant amount of preclinical data has shown the utility of PET in evaluating myocardial injury and inflammation after RT.[80–82] However, at present only a few human studies have investigated such an approach. In one of the first studies to implement FDG-PET for myocardial evaluation, 64 patients with esophageal cancer underwent FDG-PET imaging more than 3 months after RT, which showed increased FDG uptake in the irradiated portion of the myocardium.[83] Subsequently, Zöphel and colleagues[84] reported a similar increased myocardial FDG uptake following RT. In a larger study of 102 patients with esophageal cancer, Konski and colleagues[85] showed the dose dependence of RT toxicity, with significantly higher mean heart V20, V30, and V40 in patients with cardiac symptom after RT compared with those without cardiac symptoms. However, no correlation was found between FDG uptake and cardiotoxicity.

However, subsequent research has supported a role for FDG-PET in the myocardial evaluation of thoracic RT patients. Unal and colleagues[86] reported on 38 patients with multiple myeloma or lung (**Fig. 2**), esophageal, or gastric cancer and concluded that significantly higher glucose metabolism, as measured by SUV_{max}, SUV_{min}, and

SUV_{mean}, occurred in the myocardium within, as opposed to outside, the RT field ($P<.001$). These promising results were followed up with another retrospective study of 39 patients with lung cancer treated with RT, which elucidated the volume dependence of radiation damage by measuring increased FDG uptake in 47% of patients receiving 20 Gy to greater than or equal to 5 cm^3 of the heart, but no increased uptake in patients receiving 20 Gy to less than 5 cm^3 ($P = .02$).[87] Implementing PET to elucidate another interesting feature of radiation-induced cardiotoxicity, Taghvaei and colleagues[88] compared FDG uptake at baseline and after RT based on tumor location and laterality in patients with lung cancer, finding a significant increase in global cardiac SUV_{mean} in patients with left lung lesions (lower lung > upper lung) but no significant change in global cardiac SUV_{mean} in those with right lung lesions. Such a novel use of FDG-PET in thoracic RT patients represents a step forward in characterizing radiation-induced cardiotoxicities and risk stratifying RT patients, and it supports the investment of further resources in similar pursuits.

An additional point worth mentioning is the relatively untapped potential for FDG-PET to be used in the detection of myocardial ischemia in chest RT patients. Although implementation in cardio-oncologic care has not been routine, there has been increasing recognition of several advantages offered by PET imaging in the evaluation of myocardial ischemia, including the ability to assess multiple functional risk markers with both diagnostic and prognostic value, such as regional

Table 1
Summary of studies investigating the role of ^{18}F-fluorodeoxyglucose-PET/computed tomography imaging in the assessment of cardiovascular complications of radiation therapy

Author	n	Toxicity	Study Design	Results	Significance
Evans et al,[87] 2013	39	Cardiac	• Lung cancer • SBRT (<50 Gy, 4 fractions) • FDG-PET/CT pre-RT and post-RT	• Increased FDG uptake in 9 out of 19 receiving 20 Gy to >5 cm of heart • No increased FDG uptake in 20 patients receiving 20 Gy to <5 cm of heart	• Volume dependence of cardiac toxicity shown
Unal et al,[86] 2013	38	Cardiac	• Multiple myeloma, gastric, lung, esophageal cancer • RT (30–76 Gy, 2-Gy fractions) • FDG-PET/CT >3 mo post-RT assessed for myocardial FDG uptake	• SUV_{max}, SUV_{min}, SUV_{mean} significantly increased in irradiated vs nonirradiated myocardium ($P<.001$)	• RT-induced direct (as opposed to indirect) damage to irradiated heart tissue
Konski et al,[85] 2012	102	Cardiac	• Esophageal cancer • ChemoRT (45–57.6 Gy, 1.8-Gy fractions) • Radiation dosimetry, demographics, myocardial FDG-PET correlated with CTCAE v3.0 cardiac toxicity	• 12 patients with treatment-related cardiac toxicity • 6 symptomatic • No correlation found between FDG uptake and cardiac toxicity	• FDG-PET uptake failed to predict cardiac toxicity
Zöphel et al,[84] 2007	1	Cardiac	• Esophageal cancer • ChemoRT • FDG-PET/CT 4 y post-RT	• Increased FDG uptake in irradiated myocardium receiving >35 Gy only	• Increased uptake caused by either: • (1) Chronic inflammation • (2) Myocardial capillary cell damage leading to obstruction, fibrosis • Microvascular damage impairing fatty acid metabolism
Jingu et al,[83] 2006	64	Cardiac	• Esophageal cancer • RT (30–70 Gy, 2-Gy fractions) • FDG uptake >3 mo post-RT assessed in basal myocardium	• Increased FDG uptake in irradiated myocardium	• RT-induced direct (as opposed to indirect) damage to irradiated heart tissue
Wang et al,[93] 2013	17	Vascular	• Stage III–IVA pharyngeal cancer • ChemoRT (36–45 Gy) • FDG-PET/CT before, 1 mo after start of therapy • FDG uptake (SUV_{max} and TBR) assessed in carotid arteries	• Significant increase in TBR 1 mo post-RT in both carotids ($P<.002$) • Increase in TBR in aorta • SUV_{max} increased in both post-RT	• RT induces vascular inflammation, which may be an impetus for accelerated atherosclerosis

Abbreviations: CTCAE, Common Terminology Criteria for Adverse Events; TBR, target/blood pool ratio.

perfusion defect size and severity and transient ischemic dilatation of the left ventricle.[89] Although several strategies that are discussed later have been developed to diagnose myocardial ischemia before irreversible myocardial damage and fibrosis (ie, by detecting the vascular injury that

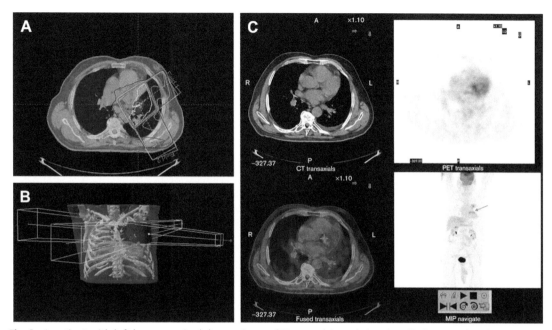

Fig. 2. A patient with left lung superior lobe carcinoma (76-year-old man). (*A, B*) Radiotherapy planning was initiated using CT images. (*C*) Myocardial increased glucose metabolism was seen in the neighborhood of the irradiation site on PET images (*arrow*). (*From* Unal K, Unlu M, Akdemir O, Akmansu M. ^{18}F-FDG PET/CT findings of radiotherapy-related myocardial changes in patients with thoracic malignancies. Nuclear medicine communications. 2013;34(9):855-9; with permission.)

precedes such a disorder), FDG-PET still remains a valuable tool that warrants increased investigation in large clinical trials.

Vascular injury

Over the past decade, substantial preclinical and clinical data have implicated endothelial cell injury, vascular inflammation, accelerated atherosclerosis, and eventual thrombosis as a causative series of events in the development of radiation-induced cardiovascular disease, with each step largely influenced by both dose delivered and the volume of cardiac tissues involved.[90,91] Because FDG-PET is uniquely suited to detect such disorders, several studies have pursued novel quantitative approaches to measure FDG uptake in both large (eg, aorta and carotid arteries) and small (eg, coronary arteries) vessels. In a prospective study of 45 patients with NSCLC who received photon RT, Jahangiri and colleagues[92] found a significant average increase in the average SUV_{mean} of the ascending aorta and aortic arch across all patients between pre-RT and post-RT FDG-PET/CT scans. These results led the investigators to recognize a role of RT in prompting development of arteritis, and the feasibility of quantifying associated inflammation with FDG-PET/CT. Similar observations were reported in a study of 17 patients with pharyngeal cancer, in which FDG-PET/CT 1 month after CRT showed an increase in the target/blood pool ratio and SUV_{max} in both carotid arteries and the aorta, again suggesting the development of radiation-induced vasculitis after RT is detectable by PET.[93] In the case of atherosclerosis development after RT, one promising diagnostic strategy could rely on the molecular evaluation of plaque rupture propensity. For example, PET imaging of plaque macrophages with FDG could enable the differentiation of stable and rupture-prone plaques by quantifying macrophage density and FDG uptake, capitalizing on the role of activated macrophages in digesting atheroma fibrous caps and triggering plaque rupture.[94]

The increased FDG uptake and vascular inflammation detected by PET in RT patients provides insight into a cause for the increased rate of thromboembolic events observed in this patient population. However, FDG-PET has the potential to extend beyond pathophysiology elucidation and could eventually play a role in the routine screening, diagnosis, and surveillance of RT-induced cardiovascular complications. In addition, further studies should investigate the biomolecular nature of observed vascular defects, a question that may lend itself to the use of ^{18}F-sodium fluoride PET imaging in order to assess vascular calcification in conjunction with FDG-detectable inflammation.

Novel PET Probes in Radiation-Induced Cardiovascular Diseases

Although FDG-PET has shown significant potential in the diagnosis of a wide variety of radiation-induced complications, a variety of molecular tracers have been developed in recent years to enhance the diagnostic ability of PET imaging. With the emergence of novel molecular probes, the number of targets that can be exploited in the identification of tissue damage has increased dramatically. This article introduces several of the newer molecular probes that have been implemented to identify and characterize the pathophysiologic determinants of cardiovascular disease. A comprehensive table of emerging nuclear cardiovascular probes has previously been reported.[95]

One PET tracer with a significant myocardial net uptake rate and a role in myocardial blood flow quantification is rubidium-82 (82Rb). In a study of 35 patients who underwent 82Rb PET/CT following RT, Groarke and colleagues[96] found a significant inverse correlation between global left ventricular coronary flow reserve and increasing mean heart RT dose ($R = -0.4$, $P = .03$). An alternative approach to characterizing coronary vessels could involve the use of ultrasmall superparamagnetic iron oxide (USPIO), which tends to selectively accumulate in rupture-prone plaques. Although USPIO has yet to be implemented in RT patients, studies have shown the utility of this tracer in monitoring plaque inflammation.[97] Similarly, the translocation of phosphatidyl-serine to the external surface of the cell membrane in a cell undergoing apoptosis is a detectable event using the ^{99m}Tc-labeled plasma protein annexin V. In patients who received doxorubicin as part of their oncologic care, imaging with ^{99m}Tc-hydrazinonicotinamide–annexin V detected dose-dependent cell death before it was able to be detected with echocardiography.[98]

As the understanding of RT-induced cardiovascular disease on a microscopic scale grows, the role for molecular imaging tailored to key determinants likely will too. However, it is important to recognize that very limited data have reported on the use of such PET tracers in RT populations, so translation of their findings will need to be verified in future studies.

SUMMARY

Despite the significant advances that have occurred in radiation treatment planning and delivery, normal tissue toxicity remains a dose-limiting constraint, perhaps most notably for thoracic malignancies. In many cases, radiation dosing and fields are based on limiting the risk of potentially fatal RT-induced toxicities at the expense of therapeutic potency. Novel medical and radiation therapy approaches are continuing to improve the survival and prognoses for millions of oncology patients worldwide, and the immediate and long-term consequences of RT are only now becoming more relevant.

The authors believe that PET/CT imaging is a valuable tool uniquely suited for the screening and diagnosis of radiation-induced complications in radiation oncology patients. This article focuses on the pulmonary and cardiovascular radiation complications that can be detected and predicted with PET. In thoracic RT patients, one of the most common complications of RT is RP, which typically manifests as an acute or subacute inflammatory lung disease. Cardiovascular complications of radiation are heterogeneous and have largely been shown to manifest years after RT; however, there is an increasing body of literature that indicates a role for PET/CT imaging for the detection of myocardial inflammation and vascular damage in the acute and/or subacute setting as well. In addition, with the advent of novel molecular imaging probes targeting vascular disorders, PET may now be more poised than ever to play a critical role in the surveillance of cardiovascular injury in RT patients.

However, studies investigating the role of PET in assessing radiation-induced complications remain scarce. Further, although not a focus in this article, PET applications to tissues beyond pulmonary and cardiovascular (eg, neurovascular tissues, muscle, or bone) remain an area with similar, relatively untapped potential. Further resources should be invested in assessing optimal methods and scenarios for the use of PET in radiation oncology patients, and future studies are needed that investigate the optimal timing for post-RT imaging and the diagnostic and prognostic value of different imaging biomarkers. Such characterization may standardize the use of PET in evaluating radiation-induced complications and allow PET to become an even more critical feature of future paradigms of radiotherapy oncology patient care, ultimately decreasing therapy-related adverse events in a growing population of patients with cancer and survivors.

Other laboratory biomarkers[99] and other imaging modalities, including single-photon emission tomography and functional magnetic resonance spectroscopy, may serve as adjunct studies to PET in detecting radiation-induced toxicities, and these concepts are under active investigation.

REFERENCES

1. Han X, Zhou Y, Liu W. Precision cardio-oncology: understanding the cardiotoxicity of cancer therapy. NPJ Precis Oncol 2017;1(1):31.
2. Jain MV, Paczulla AM, Klonisch T, et al. Interconnections between apoptotic, autophagic and necrotic pathways: implications for cancer therapy development. J Cell Mol Med 2013;17(1):12–29.
3. Boerma M, Kruse JJ, van Loenen M, et al. Increased deposition of von Willebrand factor in the rat heart after local ionizing irradiation. Strahlenther Onkol 2004;180(2):109–16.
4. Boerma M, Roberto KA, Hauer-Jensen M. Prevention and treatment of functional and structural radiation injury in the rat heart by pentoxifylline and alpha-tocopherol. Int J Radiat Oncol Biol Phys 2008;72(1):170–7.
5. Galper SL, James BY, Mauch PM, et al. Clinically significant cardiac disease in patients with Hodgkin lymphoma treated with mediastinal irradiation. Blood 2011;117(2):412–8.
6. Krüse JJ, Bart CI, Visser A, et al. Changes in transforming growth factor-beta (TGF-beta1), procollagen types I and III mRNA in the rat heart after irradiation. Int J Radiat Biol 1999;75(11):1429–36.
7. Pinto AT, Pinto ML, Cardoso AP, et al. Ionizing radiation modulates human macrophages towards a pro-inflammatory phenotype preserving their pro-invasive and pro-angiogenic capacities. Sci Rep 2016;6:18765.
8. Liu H, Xiong M, Xia Y-F, et al. Studies on pentoxifylline and tocopherol combination for radiation-induced heart disease in rats. Int J Radiat Oncol Biol Phys 2009;73(5):1552–9.
9. Elhammali A, Patel M, Weinberg B, et al. Late gastrointestinal tissue effects after hypofractionated radiation therapy of the pancreas. Radiat Oncol 2015;10(1):186.
10. Bergonie J, Teissier J. Rapport sur l'action des rayons X sur la tuberculose. Arch Electr Med 1898;6:334.
11. Evans WA, Leucutia T. Intrathoracic changes induced by heavy radiation. Am J Roentgenol 1925;13:203–20.
12. Abratt RP, Morgan GW. Lung toxicity following chest irradiation in patients with lung cancer. Lung Cancer 2002;35(2):103–9.
13. Coggle JE, Lambert BE, Moores SR. Radiation effects in the lung. Environ Health Perspect 1986;70:261–91.
14. McDonald S, Rubin P, Phillips TL, et al. Injury to the lung from cancer therapy: clinical syndromes, measurable endpoints, and potential scoring systems. Int J Radiat Oncol Biol Phys 1995;31(5):1187–203.
15. Molls M, Herrmann T, Steinberg F, et al. Radiopathology of the lung: experimental and clinical observations. Recent Results Cancer Res 1993;130:109–21.
16. Movsas B, Raffin TA, Epstein AH, et al. Pulmonary radiation injury. Chest 1997;111(4):1061.
17. Kocak Z, Evans ES, Zhou S-M, et al. Challenges in defining radiation pneumonitis in patients with lung cancer. Int J Radiat Oncol Biol Phys 2005;62(3):635–8.
18. Anscher MS, Kong F-M, Andrews K, et al. Plasma transforming growth factor β1 as a predictor of radiation pneumonitis. Int J Radiat Oncol Biol Phys 1998;41(5):1029–35.
19. Anscher MS, Marks LB, Shafman TD, et al. Risk of long-term complications after TFG-β1–guided very-high-dose thoracic radiotherapy. Int J Radiat Oncol Biol Phys 2003;56(4):988–95.
20. Mazeron R, Etienne-Mastroianni B, Pérol D, et al. Predictive factors of late radiation fibrosis: a prospective study in non–small cell lung cancer. Int J Radiat Oncol Biol Phys 2010;77(1):38–43.
21. Chen Y, Rubin P, Williams J, et al. Circulating IL-6 as a predictor of radiation pneumonitis. Int J Radiat Oncol Biol Phys 2001;49(3):641–8.
22. Chen Y, Williams J, Ding I, et al. Radiation pneumonitis and early circulatory cytokine markers. Semin Radiat Oncol 2002;12(1 Suppl 1):26–33.
23. Fuks Z, Persaud RS, Alfieri A, et al. Basic fibroblast growth factor protects endothelial cells against radiation-induced programmed cell death in vitro and in vivo. Cancer Res 1994;54(10):2582–90.
24. Rubin P, Johnston CJ, Williams JP, et al. A perpetual cascade of cytokines postirradiation leads to pulmonary fibrosis. Int J Radiat Oncol Biol Phys 1995;33(1):99–109.
25. Rosiello R, Merrill W, Rockwell S, et al. Radiation pneumonitis: bronchoalveolar lavage assessment and modulation by a recombinant cytokine. Am Rev Respir Dis 1993;148(6_pt_1):1671–6.
26. Adawi A, Zhang Y, Baggs R, et al. Blockade of CD40–CD40 ligand interactions protects against radiation-induced pulmonary inflammation and fibrosis. Clin Immunol Immunopathol 1998;89(3):222–30.
27. Simone CB 2nd. Thoracic radiation normal tissue injury. Semin Radiat Oncol 2017;27(4):370–7.
28. Epperly MW, Guo H, Gretton JE, et al. Bone marrow origin of myofibroblasts in irradiation pulmonary fibrosis. Am J Respir Cell Mol Biol 2003;29(2):213–24.
29. Theise ND, Henegariu O, Grove J, et al. Radiation pneumonitis in mice: a severe injury model for pneumocyte engraftment from bone marrow. Exp Hematol 2002;30(11):1333–8.
30. Verma V, Simone CB 2nd, Werner-Wasik M. Acute and late toxicities of concurrent chemoradiotherapy for locally-advanced non-small cell lung cancer. Cancers (Basel) 2017;9(9) [pii:E120].

31. Arbetter KR, Prakash UB, Tazelaar HD, et al. Radiation-induced pneumonitis in the "nonirradiated" lung. Mayo Clin Proc 1999;74(1):27–36.

32. Katayama N, Sato S, Katsui K, et al. Analysis of factors associated with radiation-induced bronchiolitis obliterans organizing pneumonia syndrome after breast-conserving therapy. Int J Radiat Oncol Biol Phys 2009;73(4):1049–54.

33. Kwok E, Chan CK. Corticosteroids and azathioprine do not prevent radiation-induced lung injury. Can Respir J 1998;5(3):211–4.

34. Takigawa N, Segawa Y, Saeki T, et al. Bronchiolitis obliterans organizing pneumonia syndrome in breast-conserving therapy for early breast cancer: radiation-induced lung toxicity. Int J Radiat Oncol Biol Phys 2000;48(3):751–5.

35. Gross NJ. Pulmonary effects of radiation therapy. Ann Intern Med 1977;86(1):81–92.

36. Pinnix CC, Smith GL, Milgrom S, et al. Predictors of radiation pneumonitis in patients receiving intensity modulated radiation therapy for Hodgkin and non-Hodgkin lymphoma. Int J Radiat Oncol Biol Phys 2015;92(1):175–82.

37. Bradley JD, Hope A, El Naqa I, et al. A nomogram to predict radiation pneumonitis, derived from a combined analysis of RTOG 9311 and institutional data. Int J Radiat Oncol Biol Phys 2007;69(4):985–92.

38. Kobayashi H, Uno T, Isobe K, et al. Radiation pneumonitis following twice-daily radiotherapy with concurrent carboplatin and paclitaxel in patients with stage III non-small-cell lung cancer. Jpn J Clin Oncol 2010;40(5):464–9.

39. Yirmibesoglu E, Higginson DS, Fayda M, et al. Challenges scoring radiation pneumonitis in patients irradiated for lung cancer. Lung Cancer 2012;76(3):350–3.

40. Marks LB, Bentzen SM, Deasy JO, et al. Radiation dose–volume effects in the lung. Int J Radiat Oncol Biol Phys 2010;76(3):S70–6.

41. Molitoris JK, Diwanji T, Snider JW III, et al. Optimizing immobilization, margins, and imaging for lung stereotactic body radiation therapy. Transl Lung Cancer Res 2019;8(1):24.

42. Chun SG, Hu C, Choy H, et al. Impact of intensity-modulated radiation therapy technique for locally advanced non-small-cell lung cancer: a secondary analysis of the NRG oncology RTOG 0617 randomized clinical trial. J Clin Oncol 2017;35(1):56.

43. Schonewolf CA, Heskel M, Doucette A, et al. Five-year long-term outcomes of stereotactic body radiation therapy for operable versus medically inoperable stage i non–small-cell lung cancer: analysis by operability, Fractionation regimen, tumor size, and tumor location. Clin Lung Cancer 2019;20(1):e63–71.

44. Marks LB, Yorke ED, Jackson A, et al. Use of normal tissue complication probability models in the clinic. Int J Radiat Oncol Biol Phys 2010;76(3):S10–9.

45. Carruthers S, Wallington M. Total body irradiation and pneumonitis risk: a review of outcomes. Br J Cancer 2004;90(11):2080.

46. Kim TH, Cho KH, Pyo HR, et al. Dose-volumetric parameters for predicting severe radiation pneumonitis after three-dimensional conformal radiation therapy for lung cancer. Radiology 2005;235(1):208–15.

47. Kimsey FC, Mendenhall NP, Ewald LM, et al. Is radiation treatment volume a predictor for acute or late effect on pulmonary function? A prospective study of patients treated with breast-conserving surgery and postoperative irradiation. Cancer 1994;73(10):2549–55.

48. Lingos TI, Recht A, Vicini F, et al. Radiation pneumonitis in breast cancer patients treated with conservative surgery and radiation therapy. Int J Radiat Oncol Biol Phys 1991;21(2):355–60.

49. Jahangiri P, Pournazari K, Torigian DA, et al. A prospective study of the feasibility of FDG-PET/CT imaging to quantify radiation-induced lung inflammation in locally advanced non-small cell lung cancer patients receiving proton or photon radiotherapy. Eur J Nucl Med Mol Imaging 2019;46(1):206–16.

50. Chang JY, Komaki R, Lu C, et al. Phase 2 study of high-dose proton therapy with concurrent chemotherapy for unresectable stage III nonsmall cell lung cancer. Cancer 2011;117(20):4707–13.

51. Rwigema JCM, Verma V, Lin L, et al. Prospective study of proton-beam radiation therapy for limited-stage small cell lung cancer. Cancer 2017;123(21):4244–51.

52. Salavati A, Duan F, Snyder BS, et al. Optimal FDG PET/CT volumetric parameters for risk stratification in patients with locally advanced non-small cell lung cancer: results from the ACRIN 6668/RTOG 0235 trial. Eur J Nucl Med Mol Imaging 2017;44(12):1969–83.

53. Simone CB 2nd, Houshmand S, Kalbasi A, et al. PET-based thoracic radiation oncology. PET Clin 2016;11(3):319–32.

54. Echeverria AE, McCurdy M, Castillo R, et al. Proton therapy radiation pneumonitis local dose–response in esophagus cancer patients. Radiother Oncol 2013;106(1):124–9.

55. Guerrero T, Johnson V, Hart J, et al. Radiation pneumonitis: local dose versus [18F]-fluorodeoxyglucose uptake response in irradiated lung. Int J Radiat Oncol Biol Phys 2007;68(4):1030–5.

56. Hart JP, McCurdy MR, Ezhil M, et al. Radiation pneumonitis: correlation of toxicity with pulmonary metabolic radiation response. Int J Radiat Oncol Biol Phys 2008;71(4):967–71.

57. Ulaner GA, Lyall A. Identifying and distinguishing treatment effects and complications from malignancy at FDG PET/CT. Radiographics 2013;33(6): 1817–34.

58. Hicks RJ, Mac Manus MP, Matthews JP, et al. Early FDG-PET imaging after radical radiotherapy for non–small-cell lung cancer: inflammatory changes in normal tissues correlate with tumor response and do not confound therapeutic response evaluation. Int J Radiat Oncol Biol Phys 2004;60(2): 412–8.

59. Robbins ME, Brunso-Bechtold JK, Peiffer AM, et al. Imaging radiation-induced normal tissue injury. Radiat Res 2012;177(4):449–66.

60. De Ruysscher D, Nestle U, Jeraj R, et al. PET scans in radiotherapy planning of lung cancer. Lung Cancer 2012;75(2):141–5.

61. Mac Manus MP, Hicks RJ. The role of positron emission tomography/computed tomography in radiation therapy planning for patients with lung cancer. Semin Nucl Med 2012;42(5):308–19.

62. Speirs CK, Grigsby PW, Huang J, et al. PET-based radiation therapy planning. PET Clin 2015;10(1): 27–44.

63. Rice SR, Saboury B, Houshmand S, et al. Quantification of global lung inflammation using volumetric 18F-FDG PET/CT parameters in locally advanced non-small-cell lung cancer patients treated with concurrent chemoradiotherapy: a comparison of photon and proton radiation therapy. Nucl Med Commun 2019;40(6):618–25.

64. Abdulla S, Salavati A, Saboury B, et al. Quantitative assessment of global lung inflammation following radiation therapy using FDG PET/CT: a pilot study. Eur J Nucl Med Mol Imaging 2014;41(2):350–6.

65. De Ruysscher D, Houben A, Aerts HJ, et al. Increased 18F-deoxyglucose uptake in the lung during the first weeks of radiotherapy is correlated with subsequent Radiation-Induced Lung Toxicity (RILT): a prospective pilot study. Radiother Oncol 2009; 91(3):415–20.

66. Mac Manus MP, Ding Z, Hogg A, et al. Association between pulmonary uptake of fluorodeoxyglucose detected by positron emission tomography scanning after radiation therapy for non–small-cell lung cancer and radiation pneumonitis. Int J Radiat Oncol Biol Phys 2011;80(5):1365–71.

67. McCurdy MR, Castillo R, Martinez J, et al. [18F]-FDG uptake dose–response correlates with radiation pneumonitis in lung cancer patients. Radiother Oncol 2012;104(1):52–7.

68. Petit SF, van Elmpt WJ, Oberije CJ, et al. [18F] fluorodeoxyglucose uptake patterns in lung before radiotherapy identify areas more susceptible to radiation-induced lung toxicity in non-small-cell lung cancer patients. Int J Radiat Oncol Biol Phys 2011;81(3):698–705.

69. McCurdy M, Bergsma DP, Hyun E, et al. The role of lung lobes in radiation pneumonitis and radiation-induced inflammation in the lung: a retrospective study. J Radiat Oncol 2013;2(2):203–8.

70. Jahangiri P, Dreyfuss A, Pournazari K, et al. Quantification of radiation-induced pneumonitis in patients with locally advanced non-small cell lung cancer. J Nucl Med 2019;60(supplement 1):1342.

71. Aleman BM, van den Belt-Dusebout AW, De Bruin ML, et al. Late cardiotoxicity after treatment for Hodgkin lymphoma. Blood 2007;109(5):1878–86.

72. Darby SC, Ewertz M, Hall P. Ischemic heart disease after breast cancer radiotherapy. N Engl J Med 2013;368(26):2527.

73. Giordano SH, Kuo Y-F, Freeman JL, et al. Risk of cardiac death after adjuvant radiotherapy for breast cancer. J Natl Cancer Inst 2005;97(6):419–24.

74. Mauch P, Kalish L, Marcus K, et al. Long-term survival in Hodgkin's disease relative impact of mortality, second tumors, infection, and cardiovascular disease. Cancer J Sci Am 1995;1(1):33–42.

75. Rutqvist LE, Lax I, Fornander T, et al. Cardiovascular mortality in a randomized trial of adjuvant radiation therapy versus surgery alone in primary breast cancer. Int J Radiat Oncol Biol Phys 1992;22(5):887–96.

76. Eaton BR, Pugh SL, Bradley JD, et al. Institutional enrollment and survival among NSCLC patients receiving chemoradiation: NRG Oncology Radiation Therapy Oncology Group (RTOG) 0617. J Natl Cancer Inst 2016;108(9) [pii:djw034].

77. Yusuf SW, Sami S, Daher IN. Radiation-induced heart disease: a clinical update. Cardiol Res Pract 2011;2011:317659.

78. Zamorano JL, Lancellotti P, Rodriguez Muñoz D, et al. 2016 ESC Position Paper on cancer treatments and cardiovascular toxicity developed under the auspices of the ESC Committee for Practice Guidelines: the Task Force for cancer treatments and cardiovascular toxicity of the European Society of Cardiology (ESC). Eur Heart J 2016;37(36): 2768–801.

79. Simone CB 2nd. New era in radiation oncology for lung cancer: recognizing the importance of cardiac irradiation. J Clin Oncol 2017;35(13):1381–3.

80. Cussó L, Musteanu M, Mulero F, et al. Effects of a ketogenic diet on [18 F] FDG-PET imaging in a mouse model of lung cancer. Mol Imaging Biol 2019;21(2):279–85.

81. Cussó L, Vaquero JJ, Bacharach S, et al. Comparison of methods to reduce myocardial 18F-FDG uptake in mice: calcium channel blockers versus high-fat diets. PLoS One 2014;9(9):e107999.

82. Yan R, Song J, Wu Z, et al. Detection of myocardial metabolic abnormalities by 18F-FDG PET/CT and corresponding pathological changes in beagles with local heart irradiation. Korean J Radiol 2015; 16(4):919–28.

83. Jingu K, Kaneta T, Nemoto K, et al. The utility of 18F-fluorodeoxyglucose positron emission tomography for early diagnosis of radiation-induced myocardial damage. Int J Radiat Oncol Biol Phys 2006;66(3):845–51.

84. Zöphel K, Hölzel C, Dawel M, et al. PET/CT demonstrates increased myocardial FDG uptake following irradiation therapy. Eur J Nucl Med Mol Imaging 2007;34(8):1322–3.

85. Konski A, Li T, Christensen M, et al. Symptomatic cardiac toxicity is predicted by dosimetric and patient factors rather than changes in 18F-FDG PET determination of myocardial activity after chemoradiotherapy for esophageal cancer. Radiother Oncol 2012;104(1):72–7.

86. Unal K, Unlu M, Akdemir O, et al. 18F-FDG PET/CT findings of radiotherapy-related myocardial changes in patients with thoracic malignancies. Nucl Med Commun 2013;34(9):855–9.

87. Evans JD, Gomez DR, Chang JY, et al. Cardiac 18F-fluorodeoxyglucose uptake on positron emission tomography after thoracic stereotactic body radiation therapy. Radiother Oncol 2013;109(1):82–8.

88. Taghvaei R, Sirous R, Dreyfuss A, et al. Utilizing FDG-PET/CT to assess radiation-induced cardiotoxicity in patients with lung cancer based on tumor location. J Nucl Med 2019;60(supplement 1):1314.

89. Taqueti VR, Dorbala S. The role of positron emission tomography in the evaluation of myocardial ischemia in women. J Nucl Cardiol 2016;23(5):1008–15.

90. Chen W, Bural GG, Torigian DA, et al. Emerging role of FDG-PET/CT in assessing atherosclerosis in large arteries. Eur J Nucl Med Mol Imaging 2009;36(1):144–51.

91. Gholami S, Salavati A, Houshmand S, et al. Assessment of atherosclerosis in large vessel walls: a comprehensive review of FDG-PET/CT image acquisition protocols and methods for uptake quantification. J Nucl Cardiol 2015;22(3):468–79.

92. Jahangiri P, Kalboush E, Pournazari K, et al. The utility of FDG-PET/CT for quantifying radiation-induced vasculitis. J Nucl Med 2019;60(supplement 1):1345.

93. Wang Y-C, Hsieh T-C, Chen S-W, et al. Concurrent chemo-radiotherapy potentiates vascular inflammation: increased FDG uptake in head and neck cancer patients. JACC Cardiovasc Imaging 2013;6(4):512–4.

94. Stary HC, Blankenhorn DH, Chandler AB, et al. A definition of the intima of human arteries and of its atherosclerosis-prone regions. A report from the Committee on Vascular Lesions of the Council on Arteriosclerosis, American Heart Association. Circulation 1992;85(1):391–405.

95. Dreyfuss AD, Bravo PE, Koumenis C, et al. Precision cardio-oncology. J Nucl Med 2019;60:443–50.

96. Groarke J, Mamon H, Nohria A, et al. Negative correlation between coronary flow reserve and mean radiation dose to the heart. Int J Radiat Oncol Biol Phys 2014;90(1):S718.

97. Tang TY, Howarth SP, Miller SR, et al. The ATHEROMA (Atorvastatin Therapy: effects on Reduction of Macrophage Activity) Study: evaluation using ultrasmall superparamagnetic iron oxide-enhanced magnetic resonance imaging in carotid disease. J Am Coll Cardiol 2009;53(22):2039–50.

98. Gabrielson KL, Mok GS, Nimmagadda S, et al. Detection of dose response in chronic doxorubicin-mediated cell death with cardiac technetium 99m annexin V single-photon emission computed tomography. Mol Imaging 2008;7(3):132–8.

99. Demissei BG, Freedman G, Feigenberg SJ, et al. Early changes in cardiovascular biomarkers with contemporary thoracic radiation therapy for breast cancer, lung cancer, and lymphoma. Int J Radiat Oncol Biol Phys 2019;103(4):851–60.

PET/Computed Tomography in Treatment Response Assessment in Cancer

An Overview with Emphasis on the Evolving Role in Response Evaluation to Immunotherapy and Radiation Therapy

Rahul V. Parghane, MBBS, MD[a,b],
Sandip Basu, DRM, Diplomate N.B., MNAMS[a,b],*

KEYWORDS

- ^{18}F-FDG • PET/CT • RECIST • PERCIST • Treatment response monitoring • MTV • TLG
- Immunotherapy • Radiation therapy

KEY POINTS

- Most cancer treatments are associated with significant side effects and high costs. Therefore, it is important to assess the effectiveness of the administered treatment early in the course of the therapy, so that regimens can be changed and tailored in an individual manner.
- Whole-body metabolic burden, metabolic tumor volume, and total lesion glycolysis are newer quantitative PET metrics that reflect the overall disease burden better than standardized uptake value at a single lesion and also take into account the stage of the disease and the heterogeneous intratumoral metabolism and uptake of PET tracer.
- Immunotherapy response evaluation in solid tumors is challenging because response to immunotherapy may occur early, be delayed, or be preceded sometimes by apparent disease progression (termed pseudoprogression) and hyperprogression.
- Combined use of anatomic and molecular imaging techniques (PET/computed tomography [CT]) could be pivotal to assess treatment response to immunotherapy, with PET/CT-based quantitative parameters and criteria for response evaluation is helpful in resolving problems associated with immunotherapy in a more objective way.
- PET/CT-based response evaluation in radiation therapy have several advantages over conventional cross-sectional imaging response evaluation. The newer quantitative PET-based parameters may be better predictors of response and recurrence of disease after radiation therapy and especially useful in lung cancer.

INTRODUCTION

In recent years, detailed knowledge of cancer cell biology (particularly related to receptor and cellular metabolism) has resulted in several novel strategies for management of patients with cancer. Many therapeutic drugs have shown prolongation

[a] Radiation Medicine Centre (BARC), Tata Memorial Hospital Annexe, Parel, Mumbai 400012, India; [b] Homi Bhabha National Institute, Mumbai 400094, India
* Corresponding author. Radiation Medicine Centre (BARC), Tata Memorial Hospital Annexe, Parel, Mumbai 400012, India.
E-mail address: drsanb@yahoo.com

PET Clin 15 (2020) 101–123
https://doi.org/10.1016/j.cpet.2019.08.005
1556-8598/20/© 2019 Elsevier Inc. All rights reserved.

of progression-free survival and overall survival even in advanced/metastatic conditions. The availability of multiple treatment options require continuous monitoring of patients as most cancer therapy drugs are associated with significant side effects and high costs. Thus, it is important to assess the effectiveness of a treatment early in the course of the therapy so that the drug regimens can be changed and tailored to be appropriate for an individual patient.

HISTORICAL BACKGROUND OF TUMOR RESPONSE ASSESSMENT

The reduction in size of a tumor lesion after therapy is an important parameter for evaluation of response in oncology and can be measured by different methodological tools. In the early and mid-nineteenth century, physical examination of the lesion was the main objective tool for systematic assessment of response to treatment.[1] Palpation of tumor mass to measure the size of a lesion had important shortcomings, as was shown by Moertel and Hanley[2] in their study, reporting 19% to 25% and 6.8% to 7.8% false-positive readings in assessment response using a cutoff of 25% and 50% reductions in the perpendicular diameters of lesion, respectively.

Reduction in tumor size following therapy, as demonstrated by computed tomography (CT), has been well documented to correlate with the long-term survival of patients. Between 1977 and 1979, the World Health Organization (WHO) held a series of meetings, which resulted in the publication of a handbook outlining criteria for assessment of response. These meetings were widely publicized and their suggestions rapidly adopted to achieve standardized reporting of treatment response in oncology patients.[3] As per WHO criteria, bidimensional tumor measurements was obtained before and following therapy, and the product of the bidimensional measurements was calculated and summed across multiple sites to form a single parameter to assess response. The changes in these parameters over the treatment period thereafter classified patients into 1 of 4 response groups: complete response (CR), partial response (PR), stable disease (SD), and progressive disease (PD). However, the guidelines did not clearly define the number of masses to be measured and the minimum measureable size of a tumor, thus further clarification was needed. WHO criteria eventually became the subject of reinterpretation by various research organizations and clinical groups.[4]

The National Cancer Institute and the European Organization for Research and Treatment of Cancer (EORTC) reviewed WHO criteria with the goal of developing new guidelines that would standardize the practice of evaluating therapy response in patients with cancer. In 1999, the EORTC published its own recommendations for patient preparation before imaging, image acquisition and analysis, tumor sampling, and classification of tumor response. They also formed the first guidelines for use of a functional imaging modality, such as PET, as a means of assessing treatment response. The PET radiotracer ^{18}F-fluorodeoxyglucose (FDG) was used to measure metabolic activity and tumor aggressiveness.[5] By that time, it was evident in a substantial number of studies that a strong relationship exists between FDG uptake and the number of viable cancer cells across a variety of tumors, and reductions in tumor FDG uptake could be seen in the context of responding tumors with loss of viable cancer cells with each therapy, which often preceded changes in tumor size.

Collaboration between the National Cancer Institute and EORTC provided a new set of CT-based guidelines called "Response Evaluation Criteria in Solid Tumors" (RECIST), which was published in 2000, shortly after the EORTC PET-based criteria had been published in 1999. In RECIST, tumor response was based on 1-dimensional measurements of lesions on a CT scan along the tumor's longest axis, rendering the process more reproducible and robust in the clinical setting. The RECIST criteria also objectively defined the parameters, such as maximum number of lesions to be measured (set at 10), with a maximum of 5 per organ, and the minimum size of a lesion to be measured (set at 1 cm), and this resulted in a more objective approach relative to WHO criteria, placing fewer patients in the PD category.[6–8] However, RECIST had some limitations, such as (a) it was less suitable for mesothelioma and pediatric tumors, (b) had a narrow definition of PD, and (c) was less convenient for radiologists because it significantly increased the workload of radiologists.[9–12]

The RECIST Working Group set out to amend the criteria to address these limitations and published them as RECIST 1.1 in 2008, with a few significant changes made to both simplify and clarify the criteria, as well as to allow for its application in additional cancers and modalities.[13]

In 2009 Wahl and colleagues[4] published a paper in which they presented PET response criteria in solid tumors (PERCIST), which was similar to RECIST but with incorporation of metabolic information from an ^{18}F-FDG PET scan. These criteria were a synthesis of several earlier guidelines and publications on response assessment that used PET scanning: the EORTC in 1999, Hicks and colleagues[14] in 2001, and Juweid and colleagues[15,16] in 2005.

An international working group, which included both European and American experts, reached a consensus on response assessment criteria related to non-Hodgkin lymphoma (NHL)[17] and formed International Working Criteria (IWC) based on anatomic parameters. Juweid and colleagues[15] integrated CT-based IWC with ^{18}F-FDG PET to develop the IWC + PET criteria, which was initially adopted for NHL and subsequently validated for Hodgkin lymphoma (HL).[18] Cheson and colleagues[19] and Juweid and colleagues[16] amended the existing IWC + PET criteria in 2007 and made recommendations in the International Harmonization Project for HL and NHL.

The Deauville 5-point scoring system (D5PS) was synthesized in an international workshop that first met in Deauville, France, in 2009. These were qualitative response criteria based on ^{18}F-FDG PET scanning used for both HL and NHL, and received widespread clinical adoption because of its technical simplicity.[20–23] The Lugano classification, published in 2014, was developed as a consensus of revision of D5PS and IWG for evaluation of lymphoma response and based on both molecular and anatomic assessment of disease.[24]

The various criteria for evaluation of imaging response used in clinical oncology practice are summarized in **Table 1**.

IMAGING RESPONSE EVALUATION CRITERIA

The different criteria can be divided into 3 categories: (1) anatomic, (2) molecular/functional, and (3) combined anatomic and functional response evaluation criteria based on imaging modalities used, as shown in **Fig 1**.

Response Evaluation Criteria Based on Conventional Anatomic Imaging

The anatomic response imaging criteria were primarily based on CT, and developed to assess tumor responses to traditional cancer therapy, which included cytotoxic chemotherapy drugs, radiation therapy, or surgical resection. These criteria depended on reduction in tumor size measured on CT before and after therapeutic intervention.

World Health Organization criteria

WHO published the first tumor response evaluation criteria in 1981 as a standard assessment metric and nomenclature to evaluate treatment response based on measurement of lesions on

CT. The assessment of tumor burden was done using the sum of the products of diameters (SPD) (ie, longest overall tumor diameter and longest diameter perpendicular to the longest overall diameter), and response determined by evaluating the changes from baseline during treatment. As mentioned previously, these criteria were categorized into 4 tumor response groups: CR, PR, SD, and PD. The CR (tumor not detected for at least 4 weeks); PR ($\geq$50% reduction in the SPD from baseline also confirmed at 4 weeks); PD ($\geq$25% increase in tumor size in one or more lesions); and SD (neither PR, CR, nor PD) were defined in WHO criteria. WHO has a few major limitations, particularly related to tumor measurements, which are based on SPD that result in considerable PD because small increases in lesion size may result in a sufficiently overall increase in tumor size ($\geq$25% increase).[25]

International Working Group criteria

In 1999, the IWC presented standardized guidelines for measuring response of new therapies and facilitating comparisons among the results of various clinical trials in NHL, and defined CR as complete disappearance of all detectable clinical and radiographic evidence of disease, PR as $\geq$50% decrease in sum of the products of the greatest diameters of the 6 largest dominant nodes or nodal masses, PD as $\geq$50% increase from nadir in any previously identified abnormal node and appearance of new lesion, and SD as less than a PR but without PD.[17]

RECIST criteria

RECIST criteria developed in 2000 were used for assessmet of treatment response in solid cancer and addressed some of the pitfalls of WHO criteria. The main features of RECIST included a clear definition of measurable disease, number of lesions to be assessed, and the use of unidimensional (longest dimension) rather than bidimensional tumor measurements. Defined as a CR (complete disappearance of lesion); PR ($\geq$30% reduction in tumor size); PD ($\geq$20% increase in tumor size); and SD (does not meet criteria for CR/PR/PD), with minimum size of lesion of 10 mm on spiral CT and 20 mm on conventional CT measured using RECIST criteria.

RECIST 1.1 criteria

The RECIST 1.1 was developed in 2009 and solved multiple questions that were not addressed in previous criteria, such as assessment of lymph nodes, number of lesions to be evaluated, and use of new imaging modalities such as multidetector CT and MRI. As per RECIST 1.1, evaluation of target lesions was proposed for (i) a maximum

Table 1
Imaging response evaluation criteria in oncological conditions

Criteria		Complete Response	Partial Response	Stable Disease	Progressive Disease
				Categories	
Anatomic imaging response					
WHO (1981)		100% reduction in tumor size	≥50% reduction in tumor size	Does not meet criteria for CR/PR/PD	≥25% increase in tumor size
IWC (1999)		Reduction of nodes to normal size	≥50% reduction in size of 6 largest nodes	Does not meet criteria for CR/PR/PD	≥50% increase in size of nodes
RECIST (2000)		Complete resolution of lesions	≥30% reduction in tumor size	Neither CR/PR nor PD	≥20% increase in tumor size
RECIST 1.1 (2009)		Disappearance of all target and nontarget lesions Nodal short axis diameter <10 mm No new lesions	Decrease of ≥30% in tumor burden relative to baseline No new lesions	Neither CR/PR nor PD	Increase ≥20% in size or progression of nontarget lesions or new lesion
Functional imaging response					
EORTC (1999)		Reduction of FDG uptake to background levels	≥15% reduction in FDG uptake	Does not meet criteria for CR/PR/PD	≥25% increase in FDG uptake
PERCIST (2009)		Reduction of FDG uptake to level of background blood pool	≥30% reduction in peak SUL values and 0.8 SUL units in measurable lesions	Neither CR/PR nor PD	>30% increase in SUL peak and >0.8 SUL units increase in measurable lesions
Combined anatomic and functional imaging response					
Lugano classification (2014)	CT	Reduction of nodes/organs to normal size	≥50% reduction in size of up to 6 nodes/spleen	<50% reduction in size of up to 6 nodes	≥50% increase in size of node + new lesions
	FDG PET/CT	Normalized FDG uptake (1–3 on Deauville scale)	Reduced FDG uptake (4–5 on Deauville scale)	Unchanged FDG uptake (4–5 on Deauville scale)	Increased FDG uptake (4–5 on Deauville scale) + new lesions

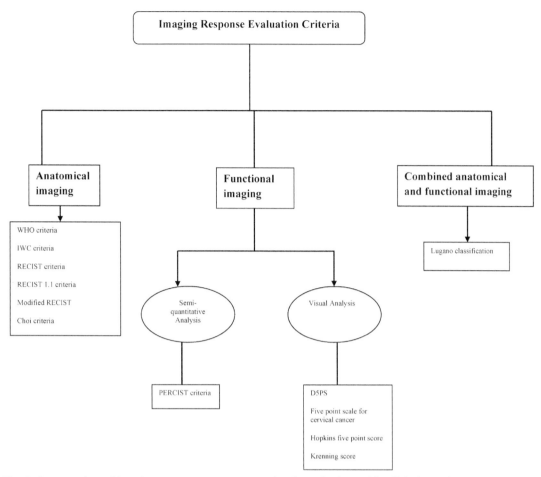

Fig. 1. Enumeration of imaging treatment response evaluation criteria used in clinical oncology.

of 5 lesions (up to 2 lesions in any 1 organ) and (ii) must be measured in their longest dimension (should be at least 10 mm in longest diameter to be considered measurable), except for lymph nodes, for which the shortest diameter is used (must be at least 15 mm in the short axis to be considered a pathologic lesion). This criterion has been widely adopted by academic institutions, regulatory authorities, and the pharmaceutical industry, and still is the standard criteria for response assessment in clinical trials. However, RECIST 1.1 has some pitfalls, such as changes in size of tumor lesions although a valid marker of response to cytotoxic drugs (whose mechanisms of action lead to tumor shrinkage), cannot be the same for the newer drugs with different mechanisms of action, such as targeted therapy agents, particularly antiangiogenic drugs or immune checkpoint inhibitors.

Modified RECIST criteria
Assessment of response rate in hepatocellular carcinoma has been proposed using modified RECIST (mRECIST) criteria, which are similar to RECIST 1.1. The mRECIST includes treatment-induced tumor necrosis and determines the viable tumor using the uptake of a contrast agent in the arterial phase on CT/MRI, in addition to measurement of the size of a lesion. CR, defined as the disappearance of arterial phase enhancement in all target lesions, which should be classifiable as a measurable lesion according to RECIST criteria. mRECIST has limitations in the evaluation of tumors with malignant portal vein thrombosis, which is considered to be non-measurable disease because the bland thrombus formed during the course of treatment can obscure the tumor.[26,27]

Choi response criteria
The Choi criteria uses changes in density (measured in Hounsfield units on CT) as a parameter to assess response, and this criterion was initially proposed for assessment of gastrointestinal stromal tumors on a tyrosine kinase inhibitors such as imatinib. In therapy of gastrointestinal stromal tumors, the tumor may initially show an

increase in size because of internal hemorrhage, necrosis, or myxoid degeneration, and some may show a minimal decrease in tumor size but not sufficient enough to be classified as PR, with a favorable response to therapy, as per the traditional RECIST criteria. The drug imatinib leads to decrease in tumor density on CT and this is considered as a response earlier than decrease in size. Limitations to the Choi criterion, however, are lack of validation for other tumors and that it is not applicable in MRI scans.[28]

Shortcomings of anatomic imaging for evaluation of treatment response

Anatomic imaging uses tumor shrinkage as the measurable parameter for assessment of response after therapy; however, this concept has some fundamental pitfalls and limitations, such as (i) with anatomic imaging there are often difficulties in delineating a tumor lesion (viable tissue) from secondary changes (necrotic or fibrotic tissue) in the surrounding tissues, which results in interobserver variability in lesion measurement leading to underestimated response to therapy on CT-based criteria; (ii) anatomic imaging is not useful for tumor responses that do not change in size early during therapy (eg, sarcomas, mesotheliomas, and NHL) and also for some chemotherapeutic agents without cytocidal effect, because they do not result in profound changes in tumor size despite their effectiveness; (iii) other CT parameters, such as attenuation, contrast enhancement patterns, and MRI parameters-changes in MRI intensity, may be better indicators of response to therapy in many oncological conditions. However, most of the criteria for evaluation of response do not take these parameters into consideration, mostly because they are difficult to quantify objectively, especially in follow-up studies.[29,30] Therefore, evaluation of response to therapy using anatomic methods in various oncological conditions is fraught with multiple practical shortcomings. Hence, there is a growing need to incorporate biologically relevant functional/molecular imaging in the criteria for evaluation of response.

Molecular/Functional Imaging for Assessment of Treatment Response

The routine use of ^{18}F-FDG PET is common in clinical practice, especially in oncology, and this is possible because of strong relationship between FDG uptake and the number of viable cancer cells, which was demonstrated in many studies across a variety of tumors. As a consequence, it is reasonable to expect that reductions in tumor FDG uptake would be seen with a loss of viable cancer cells with each therapy in cases showing a response, which often precedes changes in tumor size. A number of studies with large data are available that show that PET is an important modality for assessment of response in cancer therapy, at the end of treatment, at mid-treatment, and performed early after initiation of treatment.

In anatomic imaging, change in size is used as parameter for evaluation of response, whereas in molecular/functional imaging changes in tumor metabolism (FDG uptake) is used for evaluation of response. FDG uptake in a tumor is evaluated using 2 methods (i) quantitative measurement of FDG uptake and (ii) quality/visual analysis of FDG uptake.

Quantitative measurement of fluorodeoxyglucose uptake

Full kinetic quantitative analysis Full kinetic quantitative analysis provides an absolute rate for FDG metabolism, which is independent of imaging time; however, this modeling is used less commonly in clinical practice because of the complexity associated with the procedure, such as patient compliance issues and the requirement for arterial blood sampling or dynamic imaging of a blood pool structure and limited body part acquisition.[31]

Semiquantitative standardized uptake value measurement The standardized uptake value (SUV) is a semiquantitative method and this is routinely used to determine FDG uptake in attenuation-corrected PET/CT images. In this method, FDG uptake in the tumor is normalized to the amount of injected dose activity and total volume of distribution. Several indices are available for the volume of distribution to measure FDG uptake, such as body weight, lean body mass (LBM), and body surface area. Oncology patients on therapy usually have weight loss and this weight loss may affect SUV measurement, for example, body weight-corrected SUV, and this is because body weight-corrected SUV does not take into account of the relatively lower FDG accumulation in fatty tissues. To decrease the effect of weight loss on SUV, measurement with normalization to body surface area or LBM is used.[32] Therefore, LBM-corrected SUV is a better measurement in oncology cases. SUV corrected for lean body mass (SUL) is calculated by the following formula:

$$SUV(LBM) = \frac{Tissueactivity(mC_i/mL)}{Injectedactivity(mC_i/LBM(kg))}$$

where, for women, LBM (kg) = 45.5 + 0.91 × [height (cm) − 152] and, for men, LBM (kg) = 48.0 + 1.06 × [height (cm) − 152].

Mean SUV is average activity of all pixels in the region of interest (ROI) located in the most metabolically active part of the tumor, whereas the maximum result is expressed as SUVmax, which is a single-pixel measurement. SUVmax is a commonly used parameter in the clinical reporting of PET/CT scans and it may be compromised when images have high levels of noise.

PERCIST criteria PERCIST uses the percentage change in metabolic activity on PET/CT from baseline and the number of weeks from the initiation of therapy to provide a continuous plot of metabolic activity within the tumor. For assessment of metabolic activity, in PERCIST criteria SUL has been proposed because it shows less susceptibility to variations in patient body weight than the other SUV metrics. The SULpeak is defined as the average of the activity within a spherical region of interest measuring 1.2 cm in diameter (for a volume of 1 cm^3) centered on the most active portion of the tumor. PERCIST defined that the SULpeak be measured on the single most active lesion on each scan. In PERCIST criteria, similar to RECIST, the sum of the activity of up to 5 target lesions (no more than 2 per organ) is measured as a secondary determinant of response in the follow-up studies.

Response evaluation categories by PERCIST Response evaluation under PERCIST criteria defines 4 categories as follows:

1. Complete metabolic response is defined as the complete disappearance of metabolic activity in both target and nontarget lesions.
2. Partial metabolic response is defined as a decrease of a minimum of 30% in SULpeak with at least a 0.8 unit decline in SUL.
3. Progressive metabolic disease is defined as an increase of greater than 30% in SULpeak with more than 0.8 unit visible increase in the extent of FDG uptake or appearance of new lesions. In the absence of clear evidence of disease progression on the fused CT image, new FDG avid foci are to be verified on a follow-up scan 1 month after discovery.
4. Stable metabolic disease is defined as the absence of change or mild changes that do not meet the minimum criteria of the other categories.

SUV variation in PET/CT: common considerations The PERCIST criterion is based on measurement of SULpeak; however, SUVs depend on body composition and plasma FDG clearance, which is a known limitation for this technique. A few common errors can occur during measurement of SUVs at various stages of a PET/CT study:

FDG dose extravasation resulting in incorrectly low SUVs; failure to apply decay correction resulting in markedly underestimated SUVs; poor calibration of equipment; partial volume effects, and so forth. Also, different reconstruction methods applied in the PET/CT equipment from different vendors can result in different values for the calculation of SUVs. Overestimation of SUV occurs in contrast CT images used for attenuation maps compared with noncontrast-enhanced CT images. These technical issues must be considered when measuring SUVs for PERCIST criteria; dose activity and time from injection to acquisition also must be considered. The same scanner model ideally should be used for serial scanning of the same patient to reduce errors associated with SUV measurements. Comparison of RECIST and PERCIST criteria is illustrated in **Table 2**, with advantages and disadvantages of each modality shown.

Newer quantitative PET/computed tomography parameters PET/CT can measure the radiopharmaceutical concentration in vivo, which is expressed in Bq/mL, and this is helpful for getting quantitative metrics. Tomasi and colleagues[33] reported 2 main reasons for the use of quantitative metrics in a PET scan: firstly, metrics are less user-dependent, calculated semiautomatically, and allow multicenter trials if acquisition and reconstruction parameters are carefully chosen; secondly, the development of novel radiopharmaceuticals targeting specific tumor biomarkers warrants the use of an optimal quantitative approach. Therefore, in oncology, these quantitative metrics play an important role in response monitoring and prognosis, and are also expected to play a pivotal role in characterization of tumors in line with the development of personalized medicine.[34–36]

Carlier and Bailly,[37] in their review article, divided PET quantitative metrics into first-, second-, and high-order metrics. They reported that the metrics that can be derived directly from reconstructed volume without postprocessing are termed first-order metrics: for example, SUVmax and SUVpeak. Second-order metrics are measurements that, in addition to first-order metrics, require a segmentation step to be computed, and include SUVmean, total lesion glycolysis (TLG), and metabolic tumor volume (MTV), whereas high-order metrics required a segmentation step and additional image processing, such as tumor textural features and tracking tumor uptake.

As mentioned above, the first-order metrics includes SUVmax, which is defined as the SUV value of the maximum intensity voxel within an ROI, and

Table 2
Comparison of anatomic and functional imaging criteria for response evaluation

Criteria	Advantages	Disadvantages	Features
RECIST (anatomic)	Common use; allows direct comparison of the results of different studies Easy to use Standardized	Limited to measurable soft tissue lesion or unequivocal progression of immeasurable disease Need expertise and labor for measurement calculation Not suitable for detecting early directed therapies and targeted antiangiogenic changes Not useful in tumor that not change in size after therapy Not useful for cytocidal drugs evaluation	Size criteria for assessment of response
PERCIST (functional)	Useful for differentiating viable tumor from necrotic/fibrotic tissue Allows response assessment in any sites of metastatic lesion in tumor More quantitative analysis	Limited to FDG avid tumor SUV measurement based on body composition and plasma glucose, therefore more change of error in response evaluation Numerous technical issues related to SUV measurement result in error Assessment still based on semiquantitative or qualitative measurements	Functional response criteria reflecting tumor metabolism

SUVpeak, defined as the average SUV within a small ROI (1 cm^3 spherical volume). The SUVmax is the most popular metric and routinely used, and this included in 90% of PET/CT reports.[38] First-order metrics provide information of measurement within a limited region of the tumor (a single voxel for SUVmax), whereas second-order metrics provide information of measurements from the whole tumor, which is a better indicator of the overall tumor burden than first-order metrics.

Larson and colleagues,[39] in their article, reported on MTV and TLG for evaluation of response in locally advanced aerodigestive tract tumors. The SUVmean is the average measure of SUV within calculated boundaries of a tumor. Once this region is determined, it is straightforward to derive the MTV and the TLG. MTV is defined as total tumor volume with FDG uptake segmented by fixed threshold methods at various rates of SUVmax. TLG values are calculated by multiplying the MTV and SUVmean values. The delineation of the tumor involves use of segmentation approaches that are automatic and manual segmentation methods.

An overview of available segmentation approaches was published by Zaidi and El Naqa.[40] Methods to derive SUVmean, MTV, and TLG are basically divided into 2 groups[38]: (i) methods routinely available in a clinical practices (methods that do not need a calibration or methods that need a calibration); (ii) methods still under development and not routinely available (as mentioned by Carlier and Bailly.[37] Methods that do not require a calibration are common in clinical practice. For this, a threshold based on the percentage of the SUVmax is chosen {typically, n ε (41–70)} or SUV$_k$, where all voxel values that are superior to SUV = k (typically, k = 2.5 or k = 3) delineate the tumor. This can be done using an automated contouring program such as PET VCAR (Advanced workstation 4.4, GE Medical Systems, Milwaukee, WI) and True D (Siemens) by drawing a cuboid volume of interest covering a cancer lesion, and then the volume of interest is automatically drawn along the margin of the tumor uptake according to the specific SUV threshold. Schaefer and colleagues[41] and Vauclin and colleagues[42] developed segmentation techniques that need a calibration and are termed as contrast-oriented, which are specific to a given PET scanner, reconstruction algorithm, and voxel size. The methods in group (ii) use an advanced automatic approach with the intrinsic properties of reconstructed images and include edge detection,[43] watersheds,[44] gradient-based,[45] Fuzzy C-means,[46] or fuzzy locally adaptive Bayesian (FLAB).[47] They do not need a calibration phase and are currently under development and/or assessment.

In solid tumors, MTV and TLG provide the whole-body metabolic burden, which is the best indicator of the burden of the disease. This was validated by Berkowitz and colleagues[48] in their study on use of MTV and TLG in 19 patients with NHL as prognostic parameters. They found that whole-body-based metrics were superior to conventional indices. Fonti and colleagues,[49] in their retrospective study of 47 patients with multiple myeloma, found that, with total MTV computed with the threshold-based algorithm, 40% of the SUVmax was a predictor of survival. Sasanelli and colleagues[50] used a threshold-based algorithm of 41% of the SUVmax for 114 patients with diffuse large B-cell lymphoma and found that total MTV was the only independent predictor of overall survival, whereas, Basu and colleagues[51] addressed the issue of partial volume effect (PVE) on measurement of TLG and reported that use of a whole-body metric involving TLG depends on the severity of partial volume effect. An underestimation of the TLG value was found in small lesions, which can lead to questionable validity in the scenario of small lesions.

High-order metrics are new class of metrics in PET imaging. These metrics are used for quantification of the heterogeneous intratumoral uptake. They are calculated on reconstructed images and are referred to as textural features. Textural features are observed directly at the macroscopic level, which is great importance for personalized management of disease. Statistical approaches are used for textural feature analysis in PET scans. Textural feature analysis is a multistep procedure required for tumor segmentation, for deriving resampling of ROI content, computation of the desired matrix, and for computation of associated textural indices.[52]

Basu and colleagues[53] reported on the use of various PET metrics during the course of radiotherapy or chemoradiotherapy in 2 patients with hypopharyngeal and nasopharyngeal cancer using tumor tracking software. They calculated SUVmax, SUVmean, metabolic index (max), and metabolic index (mean) after radiotherapy in a patient with hypopharyngeal cancer and showed a decrease in these values at the primary site after radiotherapy. Similarly they calculated SUVmax, SUVmean, metabolic index (max), and metabolic index (mean) at the primary site and in 2 metastatic cervical lymph nodes site in a patient with nasopharyngeal cancer before and after chemoradiotherapy; value were reduced to zero at the primary site and were decreased at the metastatic sites after chemoradiotherapy, suggesting the importance of quantitative FDG PET metrics for assessment of treatment response, with emphasis on global disease assessment.

Quality/visual analysis of fluorodeoxyglucose uptake

Deauville 5-point scoring system A group of experts reached consensus on simple and reproducible criteria for interim FDG PET scans in evaluation of response to therapy for lymphoma in 2009 at an international workshop in Deauville, France. These experts proposed a baseline FDG PET/CT performed before the start of therapy and in the interim period. They developed a visual analysis using a 5-point scale in HL. In the 5-point scale, intensity of FDG uptake is graded to the reference activity of the mediastinal blood pool and liver as presented in **Table 3**. The D5PS is commonly used in management of lymphoma because of the simple technical classification system, and this became a gold standard for the rising trend of interim response assessment, which enabled improved determinations of prognosis and earlier treatment modifications during the course of therapy in patients with lymphoma. Currently, D5PS is applied to both interim and end-of-treatment evaluation of response in lymphoma. Response was divided into 4 categories as follows: (i) complete metabolic response score of 1, 2, or 3; (ii) partial metabolic response score of 4 or 5 with decreased FDG uptake; (iii) no metabolic response score of 4 or 5 without significant change in FDG uptake; and (iv) progressive metabolic disease score of 4 or 5 with increased FDG uptake or with new lesions.

Scarsbrook and colleagues[54] used a similar point scale in 96 patients with locally advanced cervix carcinoma, who had an FDG PET/CT scan

Table 3
Deauville 5-point scoring system (D5PS) for lymphoma

Categories	FDG Activity in Lesions
1	No FDG uptake above background activity
2	FDG uptake equal to or lower than mediastinal blood pool activity
3	FDG uptake between mediastinal blood pool and liver activity
4	FDG uptake moderately higher than liver activity
5	FDG uptake markedly higher than liver activity

From Barrington SF, Qian W, Somer EJ, et al. Concordance between four European centres of PET reporting criteria designed for use in multicentre trials in Hodgkin lymphoma. Eur J Nucl Med Mol Imaging. 2010 Oct;37(10):1824-33. https://doi.org/10.1007/s00259-010-1490-5. Epub 2010 May 27; with permission.

done 3 months after radical chemoradiotherapy. They concluded that a 5-point qualitative score system evaluated metabolic response to chemoradiotherapy and predicted survival outcome in locally advanced cervical carcinoma, which was helpful for patient management.

The *Hopkins 5-point qualitative score* for head and neck PET/CT scan was reported by Marcus and colleagues.[55] They concluded that qualitative criteria accurately predict response to therapy and survival outcome in patients with head and neck squamous cell cancer (HNSCC).

The *Krenning score* is used to grade the uptake intensity of neuroendocrine tumors on somatostatin receptor scintigraphy, as presented in **Table 4**, and primarily used as a pretherapy scoring system in neuroendocrine tumors before peptide receptor radionuclide therapy (PRRT).

Table 4
Krenning score in neuroendocrine tumors

Grade	Uptake in Tumor on Somatostatin Receptor Scintigraphy
1	Uptake in tumor < normal liver
2	Uptake in tumor = normal liver
3	Uptake in tumor > normal liver
4	Uptake in tumor > spleen or kidneys

From Krenning EP, Valkema R, Kooij PP Scintigraphy and radionuclide therapy with [indium-111-labelled-diethyl triamine penta-acetic acid-D-Phe1]-octreotide. Ital J Gastroenterol Hepatol. 1999 Oct;31 Suppl 2:S219-23.

Response to PRRT was evaluated using the Krenning score in two studies.[56,57]

For visual analysis of evaluation of response at baseline and follow-up, both studies must be placed side-by-side and need to be normalized to the same maximum tracer uptake; normal tissues should show approximately the same intensities in both studies to reduce error for assessment. These points must be considered before characterization of response based on visual analysis.

Combined anatomic and functional imaging response criteria

A comprehensive set of recommendations developed for D5PS was subsequently presented at the 11th International Conference on Malignant Lymphomas in 2011, and at the 4th International Workshop on PET in Lymphoma at Menton, France, in 2012. Revision of both IWG 2007 criteria (anatomic criteria) and D5PS (functional criteria) led to development of the Lugano classification in 2013 with the goal of simplification and standardization of assessment of response and reporting. In the Lugano classification, FDG PET/CT has been fully incorporated into staging and assessment of response of FDG avid lymphoma, whereas low or variable FDG avid lymphoma is staged with CT. A diagnostic contrast-enhanced CT examination must be included at initial staging for optimal anatomic assessment, which may be completed as part of the FDG PET/CT.[58] Contrast-enhanced CT will allow more accurate measurement of node size and better discern adenopathy from surrounding soft tissue structures than the low-dose nonenhanced CT previously routinely performed for FDG PET/CT.[24]

Assessment of response using CT and FDG PET/CT with the Lugano classification is summarized in **Table 5**. Using these criteria, CT response is divided into 4 categories at follow-up: (i) complete radiologic response, all nodes less than or equal to 1.5 cm in longest diameter, disappearance of all CT findings; (ii) partial remission, $\geq$50% decrease in disease burden; (iii) SD, <50% decrease in disease burden; and (iv) PD, new or increased adenopathy or new extranodal lesion in lymphoma. The functional response assessment is based on metabolic activity in FDG PET/CT using FDG uptake. The visual assessment of FDG uptake is used and categorized according to the 5-point scale. A score of 1 or 2 is interpreted as negative for lymphoma, whereas a score of 4 or 5 is considered positive in the Lugano classification. A score of 3 is also considered to be a complete metabolic response

Table 5
Lugano classification for response assessment based on FDG PET/CT and CT

Criteria↓ and Imaging →	FDG PET/CT[a]	CT
Complete response	Complete metabolic response: score of 1, 2, 3 in nodal or extranodal regions with or without a residual mass	Complete radiologic response: Nodal sites reduced to ≤1.5 cm in LDi (longest transverse diameter of a lesion) Complete disappearance of radiologic evidence of disease
Partial response	Partial metabolic response: score of 4 or 5 with decrease uptake compared with baseline and residual mass(es) of any size	Partial remission: for multiple lesions, ≥50% decrease in SPD of up to 6 target measurable nodes and extranodal sites If only a single lesion is present, ≥50% decrease in the PPD
Stable disease	No metabolic response: score of 4 or 5 with no obvious change in FDG uptake	Stable disease: <50% decrease from baseline in SPD of up to 6 dominant, measurable nodes and extranodal sites; no criteria for progressive disease are met

Progressive disease	Score 4 or 5 in any lesion with an increase in intensity of uptake from baseline and/or
	New FDG avid foci consistent with lymphoma
		1. New or increased adenopathy; an individual node must be abnormal with:
		  a. LDi >1.5 cm AND
		  b. PPD increase by ≥50% from nadir AND
		  c. LDi or SDi increase from nadir; the increase in LDi or SDi from nadir (the smallest recorded measurement) must be >0.5 cm for lesions ≤2 cm and >1.0 cm for lesions >2 cm
		2. Splenic volume increase:
		  a. With previous splenomegaly: increase in length by >50% of its previous increase beyond baseline; for example, splenic length increases from 15 cm (2 cm above baseline splenomegaly of 13 cm) to >16 cm (>3 cm above baseline)
		  b. Without previous splenomegaly: length increase by at least 2 cm
		  c. New or recurrent splenomegaly
		3. New or larger nonmeasured lesions
		4. Recurrent previously resolved lesions
		5. New extranodal lesion >1 cm in any axis (new lesions <1 cm in any axis are included if these are "unequivocally attributable" to lymphoma)
		6. A new node >1.5 cm in any axis

(continued on next page)

Table 5 (continued)		
Criteria ↓ and Imaging →	FDG PET/CT[a]	CT
Clinical use	FDG avid lymphoma (including Hodgkin lymphoma and diffuse large B-cell lymphoma	All lymphoma (if CT is performed for tumor size measurement); primary assessment modality for non–FDG avid lymphoma

Abbreviations: LDi, longest transverse diameter of a lesion; PPD, product of perpendicular diameters, the product of the LDi, and its perpendicular diameter (if only have 1 lesion); SDi, shortest axis perpendicular to LDi; SPD, sum of the product of the perpendicular diameters of multiple lesions (if have multiple measurable lesions).

[a] Score 1 to 5 is based on D5PS as mentioned in **Table 3**.

at the interim, with resulting good prognosis and therefore considered as negative for lymphoma.

A consensus statement by clinical experts in lymphoma used in the Lugano classification gave a unified guideline for all physicians involved in diagnosis and management of lymphoma. The Lugano classification provides a simple schema for assessment of response, which guides clinical management decisions of lymphoma treatment without the mathematical exercises associated with use of the SUV value. The trend toward simplification of response evaluation may lead, in the future, to a single set of response criteria for both hematologic and solid organ malignancies.

A visual analysis of FDG PET/CT may lead to the risk of a degree of subjectivity in the interpretation of FDG avidity. This may limit comparisons on serial scans or between different patients or centers in clinical trials. The quantified approach for change in metabolic activity on FDG PET/CT, expressed as ΔSUV, ΔSUV (%) = (SUV current − SUV baseline)/SUV baseline, has been proposed to eliminate interobserver variability in interpreting interim PET scans. The ΔSUV approach has been proposed to provide better prognostic information than the 5-point visual scale in recently published studies.[59] But this would require further validation and standardization of PET imaging before it can be recommended widely in daily clinical practice.

Comparative illustrations are given in **Figs. 2–5**, comparing the visual, semiquantitative, and general and disease-specific response evaluation criteria.

Immunotherapy imaging response criteria
Immunotherapy has recently emerged as important in treatment management in patients with advanced-stage cancer. It relies on the reactivation of the immune system to recognize and kill the malignant cells. Immune checkpoint inhibitors are the main immunotherapeutic drugs currently used in clinical practice and are broadly divided into 2 classes, which are directed, alone or in combination, toward the cytotoxic T

lymphocyte-associated protein 4 (CTLA-4), programmed cell death protein 1 (PD1), or PD1/programmed cell death protein ligand 1 (PD1/PDL1) axis. CTLA-4 is induced in T cells at the time of initial response to the antigen and regulates the amplitude of the early stages of T cell activation, and CTLA-4 blockade allows activation and proliferation of more T cell clones and reduces regulatory T cell-mediated immunosuppression, whereas PD1 is a well-studied immune checkpoint molecule and expressed as a transmembrane glycoprotein on a variety of immune cells, and PD1/PD-L1 pathway blockade restores the activity of antitumor T cells that have become quiescent. Ipilimumab is CTLA-4 inhibitor, used in patients with melanoma, and has shown improvement in survival rates in these cases. Pembrolizumab and nivolumab are PD1/PD-L1 inhibitors and have shown improvement in survival rates in various tumor types, such as melanoma, lung, head and neck, and bladder cancers. These drugs are given intravenously every 2 to 3 weeks and have been shown to produce a durable CR in a variable but a small proportion of patients.

Immunotherapy, when it reactivates the immune system, leads to the development of new toxicity profiles, known as immune-related adverse events (irAE). irAEs involve many organ systems in the body, and their management is different from that of adverse events from cytotoxic drugs. The endocrine, cutaneous, and gastrointestinal systems are commonly affected organ systems leading to thyroiditis, rash, and gastrointestinal problems.

Evaluation of response to immunotherapy in solid tumors poses further challenges: (i) response to immunotherapy may occur early, (ii) be delayed, or (iii) be preceded sometimes by apparent disease progression, termed "pseudoprogression." Pseudoprogression is mainly reported in patients with melanoma receiving anti-CLTA4 agents, with approximately 15% of patients experiencing this response, whereas pseudoprogression seems

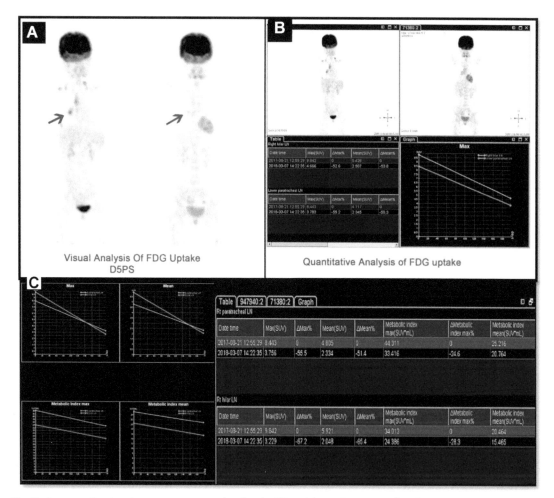

Fig. 2. Comparative treatment response evaluation in NHL with D5PS, Lugano classification and other quantitative PET metrics. A 13-year-old case of NHL, underwent ^{18}F-FDG PET/CT scans before and after chemotherapy. Response evaluation using visual analysis-D5PS shows a change from 4 to 3 score after chemotherapy and by Lugano classification (reduction > 50% of SPD of measurable target lesions, whereas FDG uptake it is same as D5PS) showing PR to therapy as shown in (A). Quantitative analysis of FDG uptake using threshold-based algorithm of 40% of the SUVmax (tumor tracking software) showed reduction in SUVmax, SUVmean, and negative percentage of metabolic index (max) and metabolic index (mean) values for both lower paratracheal and right hilar lymph nodes shown in (B, C), suggesting partial metabolic response to chemotherapy, parallel to what was demonstrated by both visual and other methods.

to be much rarer in all other tumor types (less than 3%), especially with the use of anti-PD1/PD-L1 agents, indicating that, in the vast majority of patients, progression detected on morphologic imaging is authentic progression. The clinical condition of the patient must be considered because, in pseudoprogression, concomitant improvement in the clinical condition is noted. Patients whose clinical condition is not improving and who have disease progression on imaging should discontinue immunotherapy. The worsening of overall survival in patients receiving immune checkpoint inhibitors than in control patients during the first few months has been noted in some

positive pivotal phase III trials, leading to the concept of hyperprogression, which is defined as an acceleration of tumor growth kinetics. Thus, a well-tailored set of criteria is needed for accurate response evaluation in oncological cases after immunotherapy.[60,61]

Wolchok and colleagues[60] provided a set of criteria to evaluate immunotherapy response known as immune-related response criteria (irRC), using a bidimensional approach similar to WHO criteria, and measuring a maximum number of 5 lesions per organ. In irRC, the sums of the products of the 2 largest perpendicular diameters (SPD) of all index lesions (5 lesions per organ, up to

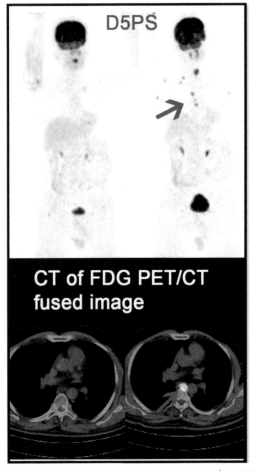

Fig. 3. Progressive disease in NHL: assessment by D5PS and Lugano classification. A 53-year-old male patient, known case of NHL, initially presented with supra-diaphragmatic and infradiaphragmatic lymph nodal disease. He received chemotherapy and postchemo-therapy, and ^{18}F-FDG PET/CT showed no viable resid-ual disease. Subsequently after 1 year, the patient complained of neck swelling and underwent ^{18}F-FDG PET/CT scan, which showed new cervical and medias-tinal lymph nodal lesions (*arrows*) on visual analysis-D5PS (score 5) and fused CT component of PET/CT scan as shown. Fine-needle aspiration cytology (FNAC) from neck swelling proved to be NHL.

10 visceral lesions and 5 cutaneous index lesions) were calculated. At every time point, the index le-sions and any new measurable lesions were added together to accurately measure the total tu-mor burden. The limitation for this criterion is that it is a time-consuming process, especially when assessing a relatively large number of lesions per organ in patients with extensive tumor burdens.[62,63]

The newly proposed immune-related RECIST criteria (irRECIST) adopted irRC set thresholds

for determining different responses including CR, PR, SD, and PD after immunotherapy. Nishino and colleagues[62,63] provided a modification in irRC in view of RECIST 1.1 guidelines.[13] They showed that irRECIST measurements were rela-tively more reproducible than bidimensional irRC measurements.

The RECIST working group decided to develop a guideline using modified RECIST 1.1 criteria for immune-based therapeutics (termed iRECIST). The same principles of RECIST 1.1 criteria were used to establish objective tumor response, and the responses assigned using iRECIST having the prefix of "i" (ie, immune), as follows: iCR, complete response; iPR, partial response; iSD, stable disease; iUPD, unconfirmed progressive disease; iCPD, confirmed progressive disease. The iRECIST has a new category of unconfirmed progressive disease (iUPD) that requires progres-sion to be confirmed by a follow-up scan.

In brain tumors, the Immunotherapy Response Assessment for Neuro-Oncology (iRANO) criteria are a set of tumor metrics to assess response in brain tumors patients undergoing immune therapies.[64]

Cho and colleagues[65] evaluated different criteria (ie, RECIST 1.1, irRC, PERCIST, and EORTC) in a small cohort of 20 patients with melanoma to find the perfect fit between morphologic and metabolical responses, and they used the term PET/CT Criteria for Early Prediction of Response to Immune Checkpoint Inhibitor Therapy (PECRIT) and included either a change in the sum of RECIST 1.1-based target lesion diameters or a change in SULpeak of greater than 15.5% of the hottest lesion in 20 patients with advanced melanoma treated with either ipilimumab (n = 17) or nivolumab (n = 3). In this study, response to treatment was assessed early (days 21–18) and late (4 months) after the start of immunotherapy. They found that PERCIST and EORTC criteria demonstrated suboptimal accuracies of 70% and 65%, respectively, for the prediction of best overall response at 4 months. The PECRIT (the combined criteria) had an accuracy of 95% and better associated with clinical benefit (CB) in patients with melanoma treated with immunotherapy.

Investigators from Heidelberg provided immu-notherapy response evaluation criteria based on FDG PET scan in patients with melanoma.[66,67] They adopted PET Response Evaluation Criteria for Immunotherapy classification (PERCIMT), which took into consideration the observed rele-vance of the absolute number of new lesions on FDG PET scan with a more robust predictive role compared with pure SUV changes during

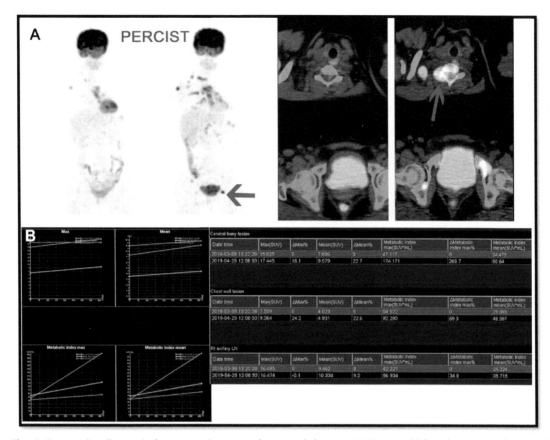

Fig. 4. Progressive disease in breast carcinoma on hormonal therapy. A 55-year-old female patient, diagnosed with a locally advanced left-sided breast carcinoma, treated with chemotherapy and radiotherapy, subsequently underwent an ^{18}F-FDG PET/CT scan, which showed a metabolically active chest wall lesion, and who was then given letrozole (a nonsteroidal aromatase inhibitor) and Palbociclib. Six months after these chemotherauetic drugs, the patient underwent an ^{18}F-FDG PET/CT scan and showed new metabolically active cervical vertebral and acetabular skeletal lesions (*arrows*) as shown (*A*). Quantitative analysis of FDG uptake also showed increase in SUVmax, SUVmean and metabolic index max, and metabolic index mean for bony, chest wall lesion and right axillary lymph node (*B*). Therefore, progressive disease was demonstrated by PERCIST criteria for response evaluation of these drugs.

ipilimumab treatment. In PERCIMT, the authors categorized the patients according to CB from the treatment (CR/PR and SD) or no CB from the treatment, that is, PD defined as the appearance of: (1) 4 or more new lesions less than 1 cm in functional diameter, (2) 3 or more new lesions greater than 1.0 cm in functional diameter, or 2 or more new lesions greater than 1.5 cm in functional diameter. The functional diameter was measured in centimeters on fused PET/CT images. They found that the PERCIMT showed a significantly higher sensitivity than the EORTC criteria in predicting CB (93.6% vs. 64.5%, respectively; $P = .004$). Therefore, use of these criteria avoid pseudoprogression reporting in various solid tumors after immunotherapy. These criteria for evaluation of imaging response after immunotherapy in oncology patients are summarized in **Table 6**.

Kaira and colleagues[68] treated 24 patients with non-small cell lung cancer (NSCLC) with nivolumab; investigated at baseline and 1 month after start of treatment. The response was determined using either morphologic (RECIST 1.1) or functional (PERCIST) criteria, along with SUVmax, MTV, and TLG. They found that quantitative PET parameters predicted PR and PD more accurately than those of morphologic criteria, and they also showed TLG to be an independent factor for predicting PFS.

Nicolas and colleagues[69] recorded metabolic active tumor volume (MATV) and TLG before and after treatment, and, excluding uptake in organs, suggested that this was due to the immune infiltrate. They concluded that MATV could be seen as the PET counterpart of iRECIST, where the sum of all lesions is used, and they found that

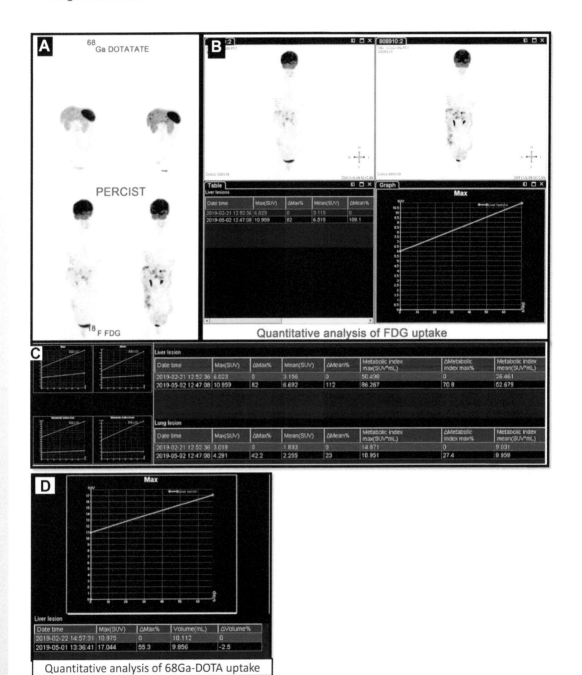

Fig. 5. Progressive disease in high-grade neuroendocrine tumor (following initial response to chemo-PRRT) documented by the FDG component of dual tracer PET/CT. A 31-year-old female patient, known case of pancreatic NET with liver metastases (Ki-67 of 25%). The patient was treated with a combination of chemotherapy and PRRT in view of high-grade NET from 2016 to 2017 and initially showed favorable response, and later on became clinically asymptomatic. A year later, the patient complained of abdominal pain, coughing, and loss of appetite, and underwent ^{68}Ga-DOTATATE and ^{18}F-FDG PET/CT scans for response evaluation. Both ^{68}Ga-DOTATATE scans showed similar mild somatostatin receptor (SSTR) uptake in liver lesions suggesting stable disease shown in (A). Quantitative analysis of FDG and SSTR uptake using threshold-based algorithm 40% of the SUVmax (tumor tracking software) showed increased SUVmax, SUVmean, and metabolic index max and metabolic index mean values shown in (B–D), suggesting progressive disease. Dual tracer PET imaging was useful in monitoring this high grade NET patient (following initial response to chemo-PRRT) using quantitative analysis of FDG and SSTR uptake.

Table 6
Imaging response evaluation criteria for immunotherapy

Criteria	Categories			
	Complete Response	Partial Response	Stable Disease	Progressive Disease
Anatomical imaging response for immunotherapy				
irRC(2009)	Complete disappearance of all lesions(whether measurable or not, and no new lesions) Confirmation by a repeat, consecutive cross sectional imaging (CSI) controls no <4 wk from the date first documented	Decrease in TTB ≥50% relative to baseline confirmed by a consecutive CSI control at least 4 wk after first documentation	Neither CR/PR nor PD	Increase in tumor burden ≥25% relative to nadir
irRECIST(2013)	Disappearance of all target and non-target lesions, nodal short axis diameter <10 mm, no new lesions	Decrease of ≥30% in tumor burden relative to baseline, no new lesions	Neither CR/PR nor PD	≥20% increase and ≥5 mm absolute increase in TMTB compared to nadir (minimum recorded tumor burden).Confirmation of progression is recommended minimum 4 wk after the first irPD evaluation
iRECIST(2017)	iCR: as per RECIST 1.1	iPR: as per RECIST 1.1	Neither CR/PR nor PD	UPD is defined as per RECIST 1.1; progression is confirmed if the next imaging assessment done 4–8 wk later confirms a further increase in sum of measures of target lesions from iUPD (with an increase of ≥5 mm) or a further progression of non target lesions

(continued on next page)

Table 6
(continued)

Criteria	Categories			
	Complete Response	Partial Response	Stable Disease	Progressive Disease
Functional imaging response for immunotherapy				
PECRIT (combined PERCIST and RECIST 1.1) (2017)	Disappearance of all metabolically active tumors and all target lesions; reduction in short axis of target lymph nodes to <1 cm; no new lesions	Decline in SULpeak by $\geq$30% and decrease in target lesion diameter sum $\geq$30%	Neither CR/PR nor PD	Increase in SULpeak of >30% or appearance of a new metabolically active lesion and increase in target lesion diameter sum of $\geq$20% and at least 5 mm or new lesions
PERCIMT(2018)	Complete resolution of all pre-existing FDG avid lesions; no new FDG avid lesions	Complete resolution of some preexisting FDG avid lesions; no new FDG avid lesions	Neither CR/PR nor PD	Four or more new lesions of <1 cm in functional diameter or three or more new lesions of >1.0 cm in functional diameter or two or more new lesions of more than 1.5 cm in functional diameter

PET texture analysis shows promising results in predicting response to treatment and patient survival. They found that FDG PET parameters were helpful in differentiating between pseudoprogression and real progression. FDG PET was also useful in differentiating between hyperprogression and real progression with help of multiple PET-based quantitative parameters.

Currently, we have no clear information of an ideal imaging method for evaluation of response in patients with cancer treated with immunotherapy. However, use of hybrid imaging techniques (PET/CT), with the use of proper criteria (as discussed above) can help clinicians to assess the responses to immunotherapy more reproducibly. Ongoing and future research, especially with regard to imaging, will provide additional information on tumor infiltration by immune cells that can be reactivated by immunotherapy.

PET/computed tomography in evaluation of response following radiation therapy Accurate assessment of response to radiation therapy and early recognition of treatment success or failure is critical to guide further treatment decisions and can impact on the morbidity of radiation therapy and survival. Traditionally, radiation therapy responses were evaluated using anatomic measurement of disease. The complementary anatomic and functional information in PET/CT scans can facilitate accurate noninvasive assessment of surrogate biomarkers of disease activity after radiation therapy.

PET/computed tomography versus anatomic imaging: potential areas for PET/computed tomography application The evaluation of response after radiation therapy using PET/CT has several advantages compared with anatomic imaging: (i) molecular response using PET/CT to radiation therapy may precede anatomic response, and molecular imaging may allow a more accurate assessment at an earlier stage of disease than standard anatomic imaging; (ii) PET/CT with specific radiopharmaceuticals allows a more accurate discrimination of viable tumor tissue than radiation therapy-related inflammation or fibrosis (after and during radiation therapy, tumor tissue may respond heterogeneously, which may not be apparent on cross-sectional anatomic imaging; however molecular imaging using various tracers may be able to demonstrate this response heterogeneity on PET/CT); (iii) PET/CT scan using various hypoxic imaging tracers may be used to predict resistance/nonresponse to radiation therapy; (iv) sometimes tumor cells may develop resistance to radiation therapy during and after treatment.

At various stages of radiation therapy PET/CT may be able to predict this development of resistance and be used as a powerful imaging modality to facilitate an adaptive individualized approach to radiotherapy planning (with potential for escalation or de-escalation strategies depending on the treatment response); and (v) finally, PET/CT can be used after radiation therapy to discriminate between patients responding or not responding to these therapies to allow early aggressive treatment of persistent or PD.

Issues in the use of PET/computed tomography for radiation therapy response assessment There are several key issues for the use of PET/CT for assessment of response to radiation therapy: firstly, timing of postradiotherapy response assessment, late PET/CT after completion of tumor response, and resolution of radiotherapy-related inflammation versus the need for early PET/CT scan to allow potential surgical intervention in the event of an incomplete radiotherapy response; secondly, a high negative predictive value (NPV) of functional imaging is required to demonstrate whether residual anatomic abnormalities can be safely monitored. This is important when PET/CT is used to guide a strategy of clinical follow-up over further investigation/treatment; thirdly, FDG PET/CT is not specific for detection of viable tumor cells after radiation therapy because nonspecific inflammatory changes can demonstrate FDG uptake that results in low positive predictive value (PPV). Also, there are different methods of reporting posttreatment PET/CT response. These include qualitative methods and quantitative criteria for response assessment following radiation therapy and, currently, there is no uniform assessment of response.

Use of fluorodeoxyglucose PET/computed tomography in various cancers after radiation therapy

Head and Neck Cancer Radiation therapy is the standard of care for locally advanced HNSCC for both unresectable disease and to achieve organ preservation. Therefore, posttreatment response assessment is essential in these cancers. Molecular imaging using FDG PET/CT has an important role in postradiotherapy assessment in locally advanced HNSCC, because FDG PET/CT showed NPV up to 99% for nodal disease (when performed at 4 months) and showed benefit over conventional assessment (anatomic imaging and clinical examination).[70] Standardized qualitative interpretative criteria on FDG PET/CT, Hopkins criteria, and quantitative response assessment parameters are used in head and neck cancer to stratify management.

Esophageal Carcinoma Locally advanced esophageal cancer is treated using a neoadjuvant chemoradiotherapy (CRT) treatment protocol. FDG PET/CT is specifically helpful in identifying interim metastatic disease (which may occur in up to 17%) after post-CRT, thus preventing futile surgery, therefore FDG PET/CT is helpful in guiding further management in patients with esophageal cancer.

Lung Carcinoma Anatomic imaging using CT scan for assessment of response following CRT does not correlate well with histopathological response because post-CRT fibrosis from residual tumor is problematic in patients with lung cancer. Therefore, the use of molecular imaging with biomarkers, such as TLG and SUVmax, to flag nonresponders early in treatment is crucial. Various quantitative PET-based parameters, such TLG and MTV, predict response to CRT and recurrence after CRT in patients with lung cancer (as shown by Ding and colleagues[71]).

Cervical Carcinoma Locally advanced disease in patients with cervical cancer is treated with CRT. FDG PET/CT at 3 months post-CRT predicts prognosis in many trials. Grigsby and colleagues[72] showed that persistence of abnormal or new FDG avid lesions post-CRT represented the most important predictor of disease-related death by 5 years.

Brain Tumors Differentiating the radiation necrosis from tumor progression or recurrence is a challenging task on conventional imaging following radiation therapy in brain tumors. FDG PET/CT has an established role in differentiating radiation necrosis from tumor progression, with a reported sensitivity of 75% and specificity of 81% for distinguishing radiation necrosis from recurrent tumor at sites of radiosurgery.

Specific limitations of fluorodeoxyglucose PET/ computed tomography in evaluation of response to radiation therapy A significant false-positive rate can be found on FDG PET/CT, which is more pertinent in patients with cervical and esophageal cancer after radiotherapy owing to treatment-related inflammation.

Osteoradionecrosis, a radiotherapy-related complication, may mimic active disease on FDG PET/CT; therefore PET imaging should always be interpreted in the context of anatomic imaging findings and clinical examination.

The sensitivity of molecular imaging for detection of lesions may be decreased when the lesion is less than 1 cm. Superficial tumors and perineural spread can be often FDG negative.

Certain tumor types, such as prostatic cancer, well differentiated thyroid cancer, and neuroendocrine tumor and mucinous primaries have a low metabolic activity, which limits the usefulness of FDG PET/CT in these conditions.

Standardized metabolic parameters and appropriate timing of imaging have yet to be agreed upon, and currently act as a barrier to more widespread clinical adoption of FDG PET/CT for response assessment to radiation therapy.

The role of PET/CT in evaluation of response following radiation therapy requires further evolution, standardization, and validation in multiple tumor types. Further clinical trials are needed for this purpose.

SUMMARY

Numerous techniques have been used for evaluating the efficacy of cancer treatment over the past 6 decades to increase both precision and accuracy in assessment of response. Initially it was evaluated by crude manual measurement, which changed to more complex structural and functional imaging procedures with the involvement of many more advanced techniques such as heterogeneity measurement, advanced textural feature, and kinetic acquisitions/modeling methods. Hybrid imaging, with a combination of PET and CT provides both functional and structural information in a single imaging modality, which greatly enhanced the ability to assess disease progression, appropriate therapeutic regimens, and form an accurate prognosis in various oncological conditions. Because several imaging guidelines have been introduced, with their own protocols and thresholds for analysis of response assessment, there is a need for harmonization so that they can be routinely used in clinical practices.

Assessment of response in patients with cancer following immunotherapy remains challenging, with a variety of peculiar aspects, such as delayed and early responses, pseudoprogression, and hyperprogression, to be taken into account. Use of hybrid imaging techniques (PET/CT) and proper criteria (as described above) can be of help to clinicians in evaluation of responses to immunotherapy.

Radiation therapy is an important treatment modality in various types of cancer, and associated with a significant risk of heterogeneous, incomplete response and/or disease recurrence. PET/ CT may be used to provide more accurate noninvasive assessment of tumor response following therapy, facilitating early adaptation, switching or termination of radiation therapy to maximize cure rates and minimize morbidity. FDG PET/CT has found useful role in treatment response evaluation following radiation therapy in a variety of tumor types.

REFERENCES

1. Gehan EA, Schneiderman MA. Historical and methodological developments in clinical trials at the National Cancer Institute. Stat Med 1990;9:871–80.

2. Moertel CG, Hanley JA. The effect of measuring error on the results of therapeutic trials in advanced cancer. Cancer 1976;38:388–94.

3. Miller A, Hoogstraten B, Staquet M, et al. Reporting results of cancer treatment. Cancer 1981;47:207–14.

4. Wahl RL, Jacene H, Kasamon Y, et al. From RECIST to PERCIST: evolving considerations for PET response criteria in solid tumors. J Nucl Med 2009;50:122–50.

5. Young H, Baum R, Cremerius U, et al. Measurement of clinical and subclinical tumour response using [18F]-fluorodeoxyglucose and positron emission tomography: review and 1999 EORTC recommendations. European Organization for Research and Treatment of Cancer (EORTC) PET Study Group. Eur J Cancer 1999;35:1773–82.

6. Therasse P, Arbuck SG, Eisenhauer EA, et al. New guidelines to evaluate the response to treatment in solid tumors. J Natl Cancer Inst 2000;92:205–16.

7. Therasse P, Eisenhauer E, Verweij J. RECIST revisited: a review of validation studies on tumour assessment. Eur J Cancer 2006;42:1031–9.

8. Verweij J, Therasse P, Eisenhauer E. Cancer clinical trial outcomes: any progress in tumour-size assessment? Eur J Cancer 2009;45:225–7.

9. McHugh K, Kao S. Response evaluation criteria in solid tumours (RECIST): problems and need for modifications in paediatric oncology? Br J Radiol 2003;76(907):433–6.

10. Barnacle A, McHugh K. Limitations with the response evaluation criteria in solid tumors (RECIST) guidance in disseminated pediatric malignancy. Pediatr Blood Cancer 2006;46:127–34.

11. Eisenhauer E. Response evaluation: beyond RECIST. Ann Oncol 2007;18:29–32.

12. Padhani A, Ollivier L. The RECIST criteria: implications for diagnostic radiologists. Br J Radiol 2001;74:983–6.

13. Eisenhauer E, Therasse P, Bogaerts J, et al. New response evaluation criteria in solid tumours: revised RECIST guideline (version 1.1). Eur J Cancer 2009;45:228–47.

14. Hicks RJ, Kalff V, MacManus MP, et al. The utility of 18F-FDG PET for suspected recurrent non–small cell lung cancer after potentially curative therapy: impact on management and prognostic stratification. J Nucl Med 2001;42:1605–13.

15. Juweid ME, Wiseman GA, Vose JM, et al. Response assessment of aggressive non-Hodgkin's lymphoma by Integrated International Workshop criteria and fluorine-18-fluorodeoxyglucose positron emission tomography. J Clin Oncol 2005;23:4652–61.

16. Juweid ME, Stroobants S, Hoekstra OS, et al. Use of positron emission tomography for response assessment of lymphoma: consensus of the Imaging Subcommittee of International Harmonization Project in Lymphoma. J Clin Oncol 2007;25:571–8.

17. Cheson BD, Horning SJ, Coiffier B, et al. Report of an international workshop to standardize response criteria for non-Hodgkin's lymphomas. J Clin Oncol 1999;17:1244.

18. Brepoels L, Stroobants S, De Wever W, et al. Hodgkin lymphoma: response assessment by revised International Workshop Criteria. Leuk Lymphoma 2007;48:1539–47.

19. Cheson BD, Pfistner B, Juweid ME, et al. Revised response criteria for malignant lymphoma. J Clin Oncol 2007;25:579–86.

20. Meignan M, Gallamini A, Meignan M, et al. Report on the first international workshop on interim-PET scan in lymphoma. Leuk Lymphoma 2009;50:1257–60.

21. Gallamini A, Fiore F, Sorasio R, et al. Interim positron emission tomography scan in Hodgkin lymphoma: definitions, interpretation rules, and clinical validation. Leuk Lymphoma 2009;50:1761–4.

22. Meignan M, Gallamini A, Haioun C, et al. Report on the Second International Workshop on interim positron emission tomography in lymphoma held in Menton, France, 8-9 April 2010. Leuk Lymphoma 2010;51:2171–80.

23. Meignan M, Gallamini A, Itti E, et al. Report on the third international workshop on interim positron emission tomography in lymphoma held in Menton, France, 26-27 September 2011 and Menton 2011 consensus. Leuk Lymphoma 2012;53:1876–81.

24. Cheson BD, Fisher RI, Barrington SF, et al. Recommendations for initial evaluation, staging, and response assessment of Hodgkin and non-Hodgkin lymphoma: the Lugano classification. J Clin Oncol 2014;32:3059–67.

25. Tirkes T, Hollar MA, Tann M, et al. Response criteria in oncologic imaging: review of traditional and new criteria. Radiographics 2013;33:1323–41.

26. Bruix J, Sherman M, Llovet JM, et al. Clinical management of hepatocellular carcinoma. Conclusions of the Barcelona-2000 EASL conference. European Association for the study of the liver. J Hepatol 2001;35:421–30.

27. Llovet JM, Di Bisceglie AM, Bruix J, et al. Design and endpoints of clinical trials in hepatocellular carcinoma. J Natl Cancer Inst 2008;100:698–711.

28. Van den Abbeele AD, Badawi RD. Use of positron emission tomography in oncology and its potential role to assess response to imatinib mesylate therapy in gastrointestinal stromal tumors (GISTs). Eur J Cancer 2002;38:60–5.

29. Michaelis LC, Ratain MJ. Measuring response in a post-RECIST world: from black and white to shades of grey. Nat Rev Cancer 2006;6:409–14.

30. Parulekar WR, Eisenhauer EA. Novel endpoints and design of early clinical trials. Ann Oncol 2002;13: 139–43.

31. Weber WA, Ziegler SI, Thodtmann R, et al. Reproducibility of metabolic measurements in malignant tumours using FDG PET. J Nucl Med 1999;40: 1771–7.

32. Stahl A, Ott K, Schwaiger M, et al. Comparison of different SUV-based methods for monitoring cytotoxic therapy with FDG PET. Eur J Nucl Med Mol Imaging 2004;31:1471–8.

33. Tomasi G, Turkheimer F, Aboagye E. Importance of quantification for the analysis of PET data in oncology :review of current methods and trends for the future. Mol Imaging Biol 2012;14:131–46.

34. Boellaard R, O'Doherty M, Weber W, et al. FDG PET and PET/CT: EANM procedure guidelines for tumour PET imaging: version1.0. Eur J Nucl Med Mol Imaging 2010;37:181–200.

35. Boellaard R. Need for standardization of 18F-FDGPET/CT for treatment response assessments. J Nucl Med 2011;52:93–100.

36. Kraeber-Bodéré F, Barbet J. Challenges in nuclear medicine: innovative theranostics tools for personalized medicine. Front Med (Lausanne) 2014;1:16.

37. Carlier T, Bailly C. State-of-the-art and recent advances in quantification for therapeutic follow-up in oncology using PET. Front Med (Lausanne) 2015; 23:2–18.

38. Beyer T, Czernin J, Freudenberg L. Variations in clinical PET/CT operations: results of an international survey of active PET/CT users. J Nucl Med 2011; 52:303–10.

39. Larson S, Erdi Y, Akhurst T, et al. Tumor treatment response based on visual and quantitative changes in global tumor glycolysis using PET-FDG imaging. The visual response score and the change in total lesion glycolysis. Clin Positron Imaging 1999;2: 159–71.

40. Zaidi H, El Naqa I. PET-guided delineation of radiation therapy treatment volumes: a survey of image segmentation techniques. Eur J Nucl Med Mol Imaging 2010;37:2165–87.

41. Schaefer A, Kremp S, Hellwig D, et al. A contrast-oriented algorithm for FDG-PET-based delineation of tumour volumes for the radiotherapy of lung cancer: derivation from phantom measurements and validation in patient data. Eur J Nucl Med Mol Imaging 2008;35:1989–99.

42. Vauclin S, Doyeux K, Hapdey S, et al. Development of a generic thresholding algorithm for the delineation of 18FDG-PET-positive tissue: application to the comparison of three thresholding models. Phys Med Biol 2009;54:6901–16.

43. Reutter B, Klein G, Huesman R. Automated 3-D segmentation of respiratory-gated pet transmission images. IEEE Trans Nucl Sci 1997;44:2473–6.

44. Riddell C, Brigger P, Carson R, et al. The watershed algorithm: a method to segment noisy pet transmission images. IEEE Trans Nucl Sci 1999;46:713–9.

45. Geets X, Lee J, Bol A, et al. A gradient-based method for segmenting FDG-PET images: methodology and validation. Eur J Nucl Med Mol Imaging 2007;34:1427–38.

46. Belhassen S, Zaidi H. A novel fuzzy C-means algorithm for unsupervised heterogeneous tumor quantification in PET. Med Phys 2010;37:1309–24.

47. Hatt M, Cheze le Rest C, Turzo A, et al. A fuzzy locally adaptive Bayesian segmentation approach for volume determination in PET. IEEE Trans Med Imaging 2009;28:881–93.

48. Berkowitz A, Basu S, Srinivas S, et al. Determination of whole-body metabolic burden as a quantitative measure of disease activity in lymphoma: a novel approach with fluorodeoxyglucose-PET. Nucl Med Commun 2008;29:521–6.

49. Fonti R, Larobina M, Del Vecchio S, et al. Metabolic tumor volume assessed by 18F-FDGPET/CT for the prediction of outcome in patients with multiple myeloma. J Nucl Med 2012;53:1829–35.

50. Sasanelli M, Meignan M, Haioun C, et al. Pretherapy metabolic tumour volume is an independent predictor of outcome in patients with diffuse large B-cell lymphoma. Eur J Nucl Med Mol Imaging 2014;41: 2017–22.

51. Basu S, Zaidi H, Salavati A, et al. FDG PET/CT methodology for evaluation of treatment response in Lymphoma: from "graded visual analysis"and ßemiquantitative SUVmax" to global disease burden assessment. Eur J Nucl Med Mol Imaging 2014;41:2158–60.

52. Chicklore S, Goh V, Siddique M, et al. Quantifying tumour heterogeneity in 18F-FDG PET/CT imaging by texture analysis. Eur J Nucl Med Mol Imaging 2013;40:133–40.

53. Basu S, Kumar R, Ranade R. Assessment of treatment response using PET. PET Clin 2015;10:9–26.

54. Scarsbrook A, Vaidyanathan S, Chowdhury F, et al. Efficacy of qualitative response assessment interpretation criteria at 18F-FDG PET-CT for predicting outcome in locally advanced cervical carcinoma treated with chemoradiotherapy. Eur J Nucl Med Mol Imaging 2017;44:581–8.

55. Marcus C, Ciarallo A, Tahari AK, et al. Head and neck PET/CT: therapy response interpretation criteria (Hopkins criteria)—interreader reliability,

accuracy, and survival outcomes. J Nucl Med 2014; 55:1411–6.

56. Parghane RV, Talole S, Prabhash K, et al. Clinical response profile of metastatic/advanced pulmonary neuroendocrine tumors to peptide receptor radionuclide therapy with 177Lu-DOTATATE. Clin Nucl Med 2017;42:428–35.

57. Wetz C, Apostolova I, Steffen IG, et al. Predictive value of asphericity in pretherapeutic [^{111}In]DTPA-Octreotide SPECT/CT for response to peptide receptor radionuclide therapy with [^{177}Lu]DOTATATE. Mol Imaging Biol 2017;19:437–45.

58. Pinilla I, Gómez-León N, Del Campo-Del Val L, et al. Diagnostic value of CT, PET and combined PET/CT performed with low-dose unenhanced CT and full-dose enhanced CT in the initial staging of lymphoma. Q J Nucl Med Mol Imaging 2011;55:567–75.

59. Lin C, Itti E, Haioun C, et al. Early 18F-FDG PET for prediction of prognosis in patients with diffuse large B-cell lymphoma: SUV based assessment versus visual analysis. J Nucl Med 2007;48:1626–32.

60. Wolchok JD, Hoos A, O'Day S, et al. Guidelines for the evaluation of immune therapy activity in solid tumors: immune-related response criteria. Clin Cancer Res 2009;15:7412–20.

61. Ribas A, Chmielowski B, Glaspy JA. Do we need a different set of response assessment criteria for tumor immunotherapy? Clin Cancer Res 2009;15: 7116–8.

62. Nishino M, Tirumani SH, Ramaiya NH, et al. Cancer immunotherapy and immune-related response assessment: the role of radiologists in the new arena of cancer treatment. Eur J Radiol 2015;84:1259–68.

63. Nishino M, Gargano M, Suda M, et al. Optimizing immune-related tumor response assessment: does reducing the number of lesions impact response assessment in melanoma patients treated with ipilimumab? J Immunother Cancer 2014;2:17.

64. Okada H, Weller M, Huang R, et al. Immunotherapy response assessment in neuro-oncology: a report of the RANO working group. Lancet Oncol 2015;16: 534–42.

65. Cho SY, Lipson EJ, Im HJ, et al. Prediction of response to immune checkpoint inhibitor therapy using early-time-point (18)F-FDGPET/CT imaging in patients with advanced melanoma. J Nucl Med 2017;58:1421–8.

66. Anwar H, Sachpekidis C, Winkler J, et al. Absolute number of new lesions on (18)F-FDG PET/CT is more predictive of clinical response than SUV changes in metastatic melanoma patients receiving ipilimumab. Eur J Nucl Med Mol Imaging 2018;45: 376–83.

67. Sachpekidis C, Anwar H, Winkler J, et al. The role of interim (18)F-FDG PET/CT in prediction of response to ipilimumab treatment in metastatic melanoma. Eur J Nucl Med Mol Imaging 2018;45:1289–96.

68. Kaira K, Higuchi T, Naruse I, et al. Metabolic activity by (18)F-FDG-PET/CT is predictive of early response after nivolumab in previously treated NSCLC. Eur J Nucl Med Mol Imaging 2018;45:56–66.

69. Nicolas A, Hicks RJ, Le Tourneau C, et al. FDG PET/CT for assessing tumour response to immunotherapy report on the EANM symposium on immune modulation and recent review of the literature. Eur J Nucl Med Mol Imaging 2019;46:238–50.

70. Slevin F, Subesinghe M, Ramasamy S, et al. Assessment of outcomes with delayed (18)F-FDG PET-CT response assessment in head and neck squamous cell carcinoma. Br J Radiol 2015;88: 20140592.

71. Ding X, Li H, Wang Z, et al. A clinical study of shrinking field radiation therapy based on (18)F-FDG PET/CT for stage III non-small cell lung cancer. Technol Cancer Res Treat 2013;12:251–7.

72. Grigsby PW, Siegel BA, Dehdashti F, et al. Post-therapy [18F] fluorodeoxyglucose positron emission tomography in carcinoma of the cervix: response and outcome. J Clin Oncol 2004;22: 2167–71.

Moving?

Make sure your subscription moves with you!

To notify us of your new address, find your **Clinics Account Number** (located on your mailing label above your name), and contact customer service at:

Email: journalscustomerservice-usa@elsevier.com

800-654-2452 (subscribers in the U.S. & Canada)
314-447-8871 (subscribers outside of the U.S. & Canada)

Fax number: 314-447-8029

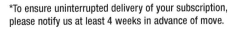

Elsevier Health Sciences Division
Subscription Customer Service
3251 Riverport Lane
Maryland Heights, MO 63043

*To ensure uninterrupted delivery of your subscription, please notify us at least 4 weeks in advance of move.